HOME
HERBAL

HOME
HERBAL

PENELOPE ODY

DORLING KINDERSLEY
LONDON • NEW YORK • STUTTGART

A DORLING KINDERSLEY BOOK

Art Editor Jane Bull   Project Editor Penny Warren
Managing Editor Rosie Pearson   Senior Managing Art Editor Carole Ash
DTP Designer Karen Ruane   Production Manager Maryann Rogers
US Editor Mary Sutherland

In memory of my father
S. M. Ody
1915–1994
with love and thanks

First American edition 1995
2 4 6 8 9 7 5 3 1

Published in the United States by
Dorling Kindersley, Inc., 95 Madison Avenue, New York, New York 10016

Library of Congress Cataloging-in-Publication Data
Ody, Penelope.
Home herbal/ by Penelope Ody – 1st American ed.
p. cm.
Includes index.
1. Herbs –Therapeutic use. I. Title
RM666.H330383 1995
615'.321–dc20   94-26719 CIP

ISBN 1-56458-863-7

Reproduced in Singapore by Colourscan
Printed and bound in Italy by New Interlitho, Milan

CONTENTS

INTRODUCTION

Despite the advances of modern medicine, the vast majority of the world's population still depends on herbal remedies to cure its ills. In some parts of the world, these remedies may be prescribed by a village medicine man (or woman) or by a local shaman. In other places, such as China and India, there are centuries-old, formal traditions of skilled herbal healing to call on. In the West, until the 1930s most medicines dispensed in drugstores were herbal and in many parts of Europe they are still the norm.

While major illnesses have always been referred to medical specialists, minor self-limiting ailments have traditionally been treated within the family, using remedies passed down through generations, just as favorite recipes for Christmas cookies or winter soups are still handed down today. Every housewife had a repertoire of cure-alls to treat the family's ills. As well as a rather potent cough cure, my grandmother's favorites included the heart of an onion for earache and a well-worn left sock tied around the neck for sore throats! Some of these traditional medicines were based on what is now recognized as scientific fact, while others had more in common with faith-healing, but it was only if these household remedies failed that more sophisticated and expensive solutions were sought from the professionals. Illness, especially minor illness, was treated within the family circle.

Today, life is very different. We have come to expect the quick "magic bullet" approach of modern medicine. Even common self-limiting ailments often warrant a trip to the doctor to be treated, in many cases, with unnecessarily powerful drugs that bring an assortment of side-effects. Ailments are treated superficially and symptomatically so that when the patient stops taking the medicine, the problem all too often returns. Infections may respond dramatically to antibiotics, but if they are the result of over-exhaustion and a weakened constitution, no amount of antibiotics will provide a permanent solution.

What is missing from the modern attitude to health is the sense that we are responsible for our own well-being. Many minor ailments are often of our own making, brought about by poor diet, lack of exercise, or "burning the candle at both ends." Modern drugs may effect rapid apparent cures, but they cannot solve the problems we persistently bring on ourselves.

The approach of herbal medicine is not just about alleviating symptoms. More importantly, it is concerned with helping the body to cure itself. It is less magic bullet, more part of a balanced approach to living well. There is nothing inherently difficult about making and using herbal remedies; it is just that most of us in the developed world have lost the skills our grand-mothers and great-grandmothers took for granted. We have abandoned the basic folk wisdom of generations in favor of synthetic drugs, which might not stand the test of time.

In this book, I have suggested simple remedies for a variety of common ailments. It is not intended as a definitive guide, but as a range of practical suggestions that can be adapted, with experience, to suit the individual. The most important first step is to accept that good health lies in our own hands, and by being sensitive to our internal balance, we can often cure minor ills before they become major problems.

Penelope Ody

THE SEVEN
LIFE STAGES

SHAKESPEARE DESCRIBED the seven ages of
man in the 16th century and traditionally,
each age, or life stage, has been seen as having
distinct strengths and weaknesses, special
energy requirements and particular
problems. Today, the borderlines between
the seven life stages have become blurred: the
"newly retired" label, for example, can apply
to people in their 50s and in their 70s.
This section includes remedies, tonics
and prophylactics that are especially
suitable for each life stage. (The
remedies can be taken individually
or in combination.)

BABIES & TODDLERS
THE FIRST LIFE STAGE

Chamomile flower

WE LEARN AND grow more quickly during the first two years of life than at any other time. Small children have far more vital energy than most adults and can often prove a demanding and tireless handful. Babies and toddlers frequently become ill in a dramatic fashion. A child's metabolism is much faster than an adult's, with quicker heartbeat and breathing rates, and a fever will send temperatures soaring, before subsiding just as rapidly. Herbs can be very helpful for babies and toddlers, especially if they are introduced to them early, so that they become accustomed to the taste.

Preventative Treatments

Caution: Take professional advice if symptoms persist for over 2–3 days. Do not give supplements for more than 2–3 weeks without taking professional advice. For dosage advice on remedies, vitamins, and minerals, see p. 83. To make remedies, see pp. 62–79.

HERBS

CHAMOMILE is very soothing. Put a couple of drops of oil in the bathwater at night, or give 25 ml of a weak infusion (use 10 g dried herb to 500 ml water).

EVENING PRIMROSE OIL contains essential fatty acids – lack of these chemicals can contribute to hyperactivity. Give 10–20 drops of oil on the tongue daily. This is not suitable for babies under 3 months.

HYSSOP helps chest problems by clearing excess mucus. Give half a cup (75 ml) of an infusion 2–3 times a week. Use 10 g dried herb to 500 ml water. Do not give to babies under 3 months and see Caution above.

VITAMINS & MINERALS

VITAMIN C should be taken in the form of fresh fruit and vegetables. If a child refuses to eat them, however, try giving flavored vitamin C drinks.

IRON deficiency can lead to learning difficulties. Guard against it with iron-rich foods, such as whole wheat bread, green vegetables, legumes, meat, and eggs.

ZINC AND MANGANESE deficiencies can lead to sleeplessness and hyperactivity. Supplements can help. Give a daily supplement containing 10 mg of zinc and 0.5–1 mg of manganese daily. Do not give to babies under 3 months and see Caution above.

GIVING HERBAL MEDICINES TO BABIES & TODDLERS

BITTER-TASTING HERBS
Sprinkle the powdered herb on bread spread with peanut butter, or another food that the child likes.

Herbs in peanut butter

SEEDS
Breakfast cereal is a useful camouflage for psyllium and other seeds. Mix them into cereal before adding milk.

Cereal with seeds

TINCTURES
Dilute the dose in a little warm water and, using a pipette or straw, make a game of squirting drops onto the child's tongue.

Tincture and pipette

INFUSIONS
Black currant or cranberry juice is useful to disguise infusions or tinctures. Add some pasteurized honey if constipation is a problem.

Infusion in black currant juice

Health Profile

NEW FOODS, NEW EXPERIENCES, new infections – the young child has so much to cope with all at once that it is not surprising when occasional health problems arise. Although babies are born with the basis of a strong immune system, boosted by antibodies in the mother's milk, they can find it difficult to cope with polluting chemicals and bacteria, and are therefore vulnerable to infection. The remedies may be taken individually or in combination.
See Caution
on p. 10.

TEETHING

Teething is a necessary, but unpleasant, aspect of babyhood.

Remedies

• *Chamomile or lemon balm infusion is soothing. Use 10 g dried herb to 500 ml water and give up to half a cup 3–6 times a day.*
• *Mix a teaspoon of slippery elm with a little water to make a paste and gently rub on the gums.*

SLEEPLESSNESS

Sleepless babies and young children upset the entire household as well as themselves. Make sure the child is comfortable, not too hot or cold, not hungry or thirsty, and that no insecurities or fears are causing the problem. Give plenty of cuddles.

Remedies

• *Add 500 ml of standard chamomile infusion or 2–3 drops of chamomile oil to bathwater at night to encourage sleep.*
• *California poppies are a gentle remedy for children. Give up to half a cup of weak infusion at night, made from 10 g dried herb to 500 ml water.*

HYPERACTIVITY

If a child is considerably more active than her contemporaries, it is worth checking the diet.

Remedies

• *Control food intake, avoiding synthetic additives and sugar.*
• *Give up to half a cup of weak agrimony and self-heal tea with a little pasteurized honey daily. Make the tea with 10 g dried herb and 500 ml water.*

COLIC

Rushed feeding may cause distressing spasms of the intestine.

Remedies

• *Make feeding the baby a relaxed process. If breastfeeding, drink weak dill, anise, fennel, or catnip tea 3 times a day.*
• *Give 5 drops homeopathic chamomile (Chamomilla 3x) in a little water 3–4 times a day.*

RASHES AND ECZEMA

Rashes can look worse than they really are. Eczema can be related to food allergies.

Remedies

• *Bathe diaper rash with heartsease infusion and apply pot marigold ointment.*
• *To ease itching, apply a lotion made with 50 ml each of nettle juice and distilled witch hazel with 5 drops of rosemary oil.*

EARACHE

Childhood earache often starts at weaning and can recur. Milk allergy is a common cause.

Remedies

• *Use soy milk formulations instead of cow's milk.*
• *Put a little infused mullein oil in the ear and cover with a cotton ball. (Do not put anything in the ear if the drum is perforated.)*

CHILDREN

THE SECOND LIFE STAGE

FILLED WITH ENERGY, fun and laughter – childhood is ideally a time for carefree play, discovery, joy, and learning. Of course, it is not always quite like that – children also experience tension and stress from sources such as school exams, family break-up, or bullying. At such times, mild herbal tonics and relaxing mixtures can be extremely

Ginger root

helpful. On the whole, children are remarkably healthy and ailments are likely to be mild and self-limiting. In the developed world, at least, few children face life-threatening disorders. Herbs are ideal to treat children's ailments, although persuading them to take bitter-tasting remedies is not always easy (see p.10).

Preventative Treatments

Caution: Take professional advice if symptoms persist for more than 2–3 days. Do not give supplements for more than 2–3 weeks without taking professional advice. For dosage advice on remedies, vitamins, and minerals, see p. 83. To make remedies, see pp. 62–79.

— HERBS —

GINGER is a pleasant-tasting herb. It combats motion sickness, provides a warming remedy for colds and chills, and is soothing for digestive upsets. Give in the form of crystallized ginger or ginger cookies, as an alternative to ginger capsules.

LICORICE is helpful for constipation, and children usually like its sweet taste. Give 10 drops of fluid extract up to 3 times a day.

SESAME SEEDS are rich in calcium and other minerals and provide a nutritious addition to the diet. Use them in cooking, on salads, and with breakfast cereals.

— VITAMINS & MINERALS —

MAGNESIUM deficiency can cause muscle cramps, poor appetite, sleeplessness, and behavioral problems. Give a daily supplement containing up to 800 mg.

ZINC deficiency is common in childhood and has been implicated in a wide range of problems, including dyslexia, growth problems, leg pains, and insomnia. Give a daily supplement containing up to 50 mg.

B VITAMIN deficiencies, especially B_1 and B_6, can lead to restlessness, fatigue, and learning difficulties. Make sure the child is eating a healthy diet and give a daily supplement containing 10–20 mg of B_1 and 1–2 mg of B_6.

TIMELY TONICS

AMERICAN GINSENG
A gentle, but strengthening tonic, that suits children exhausted at the end of school or worn down by infections. Give 10 drops of tincture in a little water daily. *Tincture*

SHU DI HUANG
A traditional Chinese childhood tonic, this herb strengthens growing bones and tissues. Give 10 drops of tincture in a little warm water daily.

Tincture

GOTU KOLA
This Indian herb can be helpful for hyperactive children. Give a daily cup of infusion made with 15 g herb to 500 ml water.

Dried herb

SESAME OIL
Massage with warm sesame oil helps emotional upsets. Add 4 drops of lavender oil to 10 ml sesame oil and gently massage the shoulders and abdomen.

Oil

Health Profile

SCHOOL IS NOT JUST the place where children learn, it is also where they pick up infections and infestations, such as chickenpox, colds, and head lice. Keeping children healthy, by making sure they eat well and get plenty of fresh air, can help them combat such attacks. It also helps to limit their reliance on antibiotics, thereby avoiding immune system problems in later life.

NITS

Head lice are common in schools. Check for eggs on the scalp, at the nape of the neck.

Remedies

• *Put tea tree oil on a fine-toothed comb and comb the hair thoroughly weekly, until the problem clears.*
• *Add 5 ml each of thyme and tea tree oils to 250 ml ordinary shampoo. Use to wash hair 2–3 times a week.*

COLDS AND INFECTIONS

All day in an airless classroom, followed by hours playing computer games, is a sure way to encourage stuffy heads and infections. Children's immune systems are usually strong, but recurring colds and repeated use of antibiotics soon weaken them.

Remedies

• *Give a cup of catnip infusion made with 20 g herb to 500 ml water, flavored with a little honey or peppermint essence to help combat chills and congestion.*
• *Give 10–20 drops of echinacea tincture in fruit juice daily to boost the immune system and combat infection.*

UPSET TUMMIES AND DIARRHEA

Excitement, overeating, tension, and antibiotics can all lead to digestive upsets or diarrhea. Biliousness – attacks of nausea and vomiting – in childhood can be a forerunner of migraine in later life and may be linked to food sensitivities.

Remedies

• *Give plenty of fluids for diarrhea – try black currant or cranberry juice.*
• *For nausea and chronic diarrhea, give a cup of ginger root decoction, (use 20 g root to 600 ml water).*
• *Give a runny paste with 2 teaspoons of powdered slippery elm in hot water to soothe the stomach. Add yogurt to make it more palatable.*
• *For problems related to over-excitement, stress, or food sensitivities, give a cup of lemon balm and agrimony tea made with 10 g of each herb to 500 ml water*

BEDWETTING

Anxiety, infections, and inherited tendencies can all cause bedwetting. Lots of cuddles and affection may be needed if the problem is related to insecurity, caused by changing schools or moving house.

Remedies

• *Give 5–10 drops of sweet sumach or St.-John's-wort tincture in warm water about 20 minutes before bed.*
• *For infections or bladder irritations, give a cup of buchu and cornsilk tea, made with 5 g of each herb and 200 ml water, 90 minutes before bedtime. Flavor with black currant juice if desired.*

CUTS AND SCRATCHES

Cuts and scratches are an inevitable part of childhood. Keep them clean and discourage children from picking the scabs.

Remedies

• *Add 5 ml of marigold tincture to 500 ml boiled water and bathe cuts from the center outward before applying a dressing or bandage.*
• *Use pot marigold or St.-John's-wort cream on cuts and broken skin.*

ADOLESCENTS

THE THIRD LIFE STAGE

FOR BOTH SEXES, adolescence is a time of rapid physical and mental change. It is also an age for establishing self-confidence and forging a new adult identity. For some, this means a period of difficult and rebellious behavior that may cause discord within the family. Testing the waters of adulthood usually involves experimentation – ranging

Marigold flower

from trying out different clothes and hairstyles, to drinking alcohol, smoking, having sex, and abusing drugs. Luckily, most people survive this life stage unscathed and emerge, a little wiser, into young adulthood. Helpful remedies include Bach Flower Remedies to ease mood swings and tonics such as dandelion that cleanse the system.

Preventative Treatments

A healthy diet should be sufficient, but the following supplements may be useful during the growth spurts of adolescence. For dosage advice on remedies, vitamins, and minerals, see p. 83. For instructions on making remedies, see pp. 62–79.

HERBS

POT MARIGOLD is antifungal and antiseptic. Rub the cream regularly onto the face to help prevent pimples.

ALFALFA is an excellent source of vitamins and minerals, which are often missing from the junk food loved by teenagers. Use the sprouted seeds in sandwiches or as a garnish for omelets and burgers.

DANDELION is a good liver tonic and cleansing herb, important for anyone exposed to synthetic chemicals, including food additives or those found in a polluted atmosphere. Take dandelion root as a decoction or use dandelion root coffee substitutes.

VITAMINS & MINERALS

CALCIUM is found in dairy products, green vegetables, nuts, seeds, and legumes, and a healthy diet usually ensures an adequate supply. Calcium requirements are higher during growth periods, so try eating more of these foods or take up to 250 mg daily.

ZINC is important for hormonal development. Boost intake by eating more meat, nuts, egg yolk, legumes, and pumpkin seeds, or take up to 50 mg daily.

VITAMIN B₂ (riboflavin) requirements increase at times of rapid growth. Eat plenty of dairy products, cereals, and meat, or take 5–20 mg daily.

TIMELY TONICS

ROSEMARY
A stimulant tonic traditionally believed to improve the memory. Take a cup of standard infusion daily to improve concentration.

Dried herb

CINNAMON
A warming tonic that is helpful during the hormonal changes and growth spurts of puberty. Try sprinkling the powder on hot buttered toast.

Cinnamon on toast

STINGING NETTLE
An ideal nutritional boost for a junk-food diet. Take 3 x 200 mg capsules or 10 ml juice daily.

Capsules

BAI ZHI
To regulate the appetite, take 20 drops tincture in warm water daily. For anorexia, mix with an equal amount of Chen Pi and take 2 x 200 mg capsules 3 times daily.

Capsules

Health Profile

IRREGULAR MEALS, alcohol, late nights: the adolescent is almost asking for problems. Luckily, most teenagers are extremely healthy, although burning the candle at both ends leads to increased risk of infection and infectious mononucleosis. Others may become obsessed with dieting and succumb to eating disorders such as anorexia.

ACNE

Teenage pimples can become a major preoccupation. The cause is likely to be poor diet. In girls they can be linked to menstrual imbalances, becoming worse before a period.

Remedies

• *Rubbing a garlic clove on pimples at night or washing in water in which cabbage has been boiled may not sound appealing, but both are effective treatments.*
• *Make a lotion with 30 ml each of pot marigold tincture, distilled witch hazel, and rose water with 5 ml of tea tree oil. Apply with a cotton ball 2–3 times daily.*

INFECTIOUS MONONUCLEOSIS

Infectious mononucleosis occurs commonly among adolescents and young adults. It starts with a sore throat, listlessness, and aching muscles. Enlarged, tender glands can linger for up to 4 months.

Remedies

• *During the acute, early stages, take 5–10 ml each of echinacea and cleavers tincture 3–4 times a day.*
• *During convalescence, mix equal amounts of Siberian ginseng, oats, and vervain tinctures, and take 5 ml 4 times daily. Add a few drops of wormwood tincture to improve the appetite and aid digestion.*

IRREGULAR OR PAINFUL PERIODS

It often takes 2 or 3 years for a young girl's periods to settle down after puberty and establish a pattern.

Remedies

• *A daily cup of standard infusion of St.-John's-wort can help relaxation and ease pain.*
• *Take 20 ml of black haw bark tincture when period cramps start: repeat if necessary after 4 hours.*

MOODINESS AND IRRITABILITY

Mood swings, ranging from euphoria to depression and tears, are commonplace, as teenagers cope with the trials and tribulations of growing up.

Remedies

• *Bach Flower Remedies can be especially helpful; try vervain for feelings of injustice and holly to combat anger and hatred. Take 2 drops of each diluted in 20 ml of water at frequent intervals.*
• *Add 2–3 drops of sandalwood and lavender oil to bathwater at night to aid relaxation.*

FOOD FADS

Adolescents are especially prone to eating disorders, special diets, or meat aversion, and in all cases nutritional balance may become upset. Caution. Professional help for eating disorders is vital.

Remedies

• *Vegetarians should eat legumes and grains at each meal. Vegans should take 50 μg of vitamin B_{12}.*
• *To stimulate the appetite, take 2–5 drops tincture of a digestive stimulant such as barberry, in a little warm water before meals.*
• *If tension is adding to the problem, drink a cup of standard infusion of a relaxing nervine, such as chamomile.*

YOUNG WORKING PEOPLE
THE FOURTH LIFE STAGE

LIFE IS BUSY for people in their 20s and 30s and good health is often taken for granted. Minor ailments are usually shrugged off fairly easily, while more serious conditions are frequently ignored. Maintaining a healthy lifestyle can be difficult when you rush or miss meals, have little time to relax and unwind, consume an excess of alcohol, and smoke cigarettes. But neglect and over-

Echinacea flower

indulgence at this stage can lead to long-term problems, as ignored sprains and strains sow the seeds of arthritis, for example, while persistent gastritis can develop into ulcers. Herbs can be used to treat the common, self-limiting problems of healthy adults, and they are also useful as gentle tonics – soothing stresses and providing energy to help the system cope with peaks of activity.

Preventative Treatments

A healthy diet is essential, but some of the following may help in times of stress. See p. 126 for herbs to avoid in pregnancy.
For dosage advice on remedies, vitamins, and minerals, see p. 83. For instructions on making remedies, see pp. 62–79.

HERBS

ECHINACEA boosts the immune system. At the first hint of colds or flu or if suffering from stress, take 3 x 200 mg capsules 3 times a day.

MILK THISTLE SEEDS are a good restorative for the liver, especially if alcohol intake is high. Take 5 ml of tincture before heading for the party – and again first thing next morning (and don't drink to excess).

CLEAVERS cleanse the lymphatic system. Take 5–10 ml of tincture or pulp ten cups of fresh herb in a food processor to make a thick green drink. Take 3 times daily.

VITAMINS & MINERALS

B VITAMINS are often deficient if the diet is poor, if alcohol consumption is high, or if long-term medication is being taken (including oral contraceptives). Take 400–800 mg vitamin B complex daily.

VITAMIN C helps those prone to infections. Eat plenty of fruit or take 500-1,000 mg per day. Heavy smokers can benefit from high doses (up to 3 g per day).

ZINC absorption can be affected by high alcohol intake, or low protein consumption. Eat plenty of nuts, legumes, and whole wheat bread, or take up to 50 mg a day.

TIMELY TONICS

ASTRAGALUS ROOT
This is an effective energy tonic, popular in China with young adults. Take 1–2 x 200 mg capsules or a sherry glass of tonic wine daily.

Tonic wine

HE SHOU WU
The Chinese believe this helps to increase reproductive energy. Take a sherry glass of tonic wine daily.

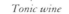

Tonic wine

SCHIZANDRA FRUIT
An aphrodisiac for both men and women, this herb also improves ability to cope with stress. Take 2 x 200 mg capsules or a sherry glass of tonic wine daily.

Dried fruit

SIBERIAN GINSENG
An excellent remedy to increase stamina and help the system cope with stress. Take 3 x 200 mg capsules or tablets daily.

Tablets

Health Profile

LIVING LIFE to its fullest may bring problems of excess. Too much alcohol, junk food, nicotine, or caffeine combined with too little exercise or relaxation can soon lead to minor health problems such as gastritis and minor headaches, which if neglected will only get worse. It is essential to eat a balanced diet and try to adopt a healthy lifestyle during this life stage as an investment for later years.

GASTRITIS
Too much alcohol and contaminated food – often inadequately reheated in a microwave – are common causes of acute gastritis, characterized by vomiting and diarrhea lasting for 1–2 days.

Remedies
• *Cold Indian tea without milk or sugar can help reduce gut inflammation and ease symptoms.*
• *Take 2–3 slippery elm capsules every 3–4 hours, or mix a teaspoon of slippery elm powder in a cup of hot water and drink every 3–4 hours while symptoms persist.*

SPRAINED JOINTS AND MUSCLES
Sports and exercise, such as squash, football, tennis, and jogging can cause joint injuries, which if not remedied in youth can all too easily lead to arthritis in old age.

Remedies
• *Use elastic tubular bandages to support sprained ankles.*
• *For sprains and strains, mix 5 drops each of rosemary, thyme, sage, and lavender oils with 10 ml sweet almond oil and rub in twice a day.*
• *Use arnica cream on bruises and sprains and take a homeopathic Arnica 6x tablet every 4 hours after painful accidents.*

TENSION HEADACHES
Long working hours, deadlines, a stressful journey home and too much caffeine can all cause tension headaches. Learning to relax is an essential part of treatment.

Remedies
• *Mix 5 drops of lavender oil in 5 ml of sweet almond oil and massage the temples and neck.*
• *Drink a cup of chamomile and wood betony infusion for relaxation. (Note: Avoid wood betony in pregnancy.)*

ULCERATIVE COLITIS
Excessive and recurrent diarrhea and depression are the hallmarks of this debilitating condition that is most common among young adults. It is often stress-related and can be worse in pregnancy.

Remedies
• *Drink a cup of chamomile and agrimony infusion 3–6 times daily.*
• *Take 2–3 capsules of slippery elm 3 times a day or chew a small piece of licorice stick once or twice a day to ease inflammation.*

PREMENSTRUAL SYNDROME
Too much coffee or chocolate, and an irregular or worrying sex life can contribute to pre-menstrual tension, which is often severe in young, childless women. Avoiding artificial stimulants and getting exercise can help.

Remedies
• *Take a cup of Dang Gui (Chinese angelica) decoction daily.*
• *Try 10–20 drops of chaste-tree tincture in water each morning.*
• *Take 500 mg of evening primrose supplements daily.*
• *Vitamin B$_6$ can be helpful in some cases. Take 2–10 mg daily, preferably in a B-complex mix.*

PARENTHOOD

—— THE FOURTH LIFE STAGE ——

WHETHER FROM preference or financial necessity, young parents frequently combine full-time jobs with the demands of small children, often with very little outside help. In the past, grandparents were usually on hand to help with childcare, but today they may live miles away and be fully occupied with their own lives. For many people, the arrival of children, with the inevitable

Lemon balm leaves

pressures on time and finances, marks a decline in their social life and can lead to a growing dissatisfaction with the demands of a young family. Personal interests may become neglected, so it is important for parents to schedule "private time" alone together. Herbs can help encourage relaxation for the parents, thereby reducing tensions for the whole family.

Preventative Treatments

No one who is young and fit should take too many supplements, but a few of these may be useful. See p. 126 for herbs to avoid during pregnancy. For dosage advice on remedies, vitamins, and minerals, see p. 83. For instructions on making remedies, see pp. 62–79.

—— HERBS ——

LEMON BALM soothes the digestion, and is a good antidepressant, helpful for postnatal problems. Drink a cup of standard infusion daily.

LINDEN FLOWERS calm stressed nerves and reduce the risk of atherosclerosis (hardening of the arteries). Take a cup of standard infusion 2–3 times daily, flavored with a little peppermint.

EVENING PRIMROSE OIL contains essential fatty acids and can ease menstrual irregularities. Take a daily supplement of 250–500 mg for several months.

—— VITAMINS & MINERALS ——

VITAMIN E can help lower raised cholesterol levels, especially in young adults. Take 300–600 IUs daily.

MAGNESIUM levels are sometimes low in premenstrual tension sufferers, particularly if the diet is poor. Take 400–800 mg daily.

IRON intake of vegetarians and menstruating women is often insufficient. Eat plenty of whole wheat bread, legumes, egg yolk, parsley, watercress, and (if not vegetarian) shellfish, liver, and kidney. Alternatively, take up to 40 mg daily.

TIMELY TONICS

DANG GUI
A tonic for the female reproductive system and helpful for anemia. Take tablets (follow the dosage instructions on the package). Do not take during pregnancy.

Tablets

MARJORAM OIL
Use 2–3 drops in baths to counter stress or tiredness, or add 5 drops to 5 ml of sweet almond oil and use as a massage oil. (Do not use during pregnancy.)

Oil

ROYAL JELLY
A traditional tonic, also now believed to improve female fertility. It provides many vitamins and amino acids. Take 1–2 x 250 mg capsules or a 10 ml phial daily.

Capsules

GAN CAO
An excellent energy tonic and detoxifier. Chew small pieces of root or take a sherry glass of tonic wine daily. (Do not take if suffering from high blood pressure.)

Tonic wine

Health Profile

"DON'T PANIC" SHOULD be the motto of every young family, as financial crises loom and toddlers wreak havoc and succumb to endless infections. Regular relaxation is important for both parents, since a buildup of stress can all too often pave the way for nervous disorders and long-term physical problems.

IRRITABILITY

Children can be hard work and test the patience of a saint. Learn to ignore minor irritations and find time for a little personal pampering.

Remedies
• *Drink an infusion of wood betony regularly instead of tea or coffee. (Avoid in pregnancy.)*
• *Add 2–3 drops of lavender or geranium oils to bathwater to soothe frayed nerves.*
• *Try Bach Flower Remedies – beech to ease intolerance and impatiens for general irritability. Add red chestnut for worry or elm for inability to cope.*

LOSS OF LIBIDO

Exhaustion frequently take its toll on a couple's sex life, and it is important to spend time relaxing together.

Remedies
• *Burn a few drops of jasmine and sandalwood oils in a diffuser attached to an electric lamp.*
• *Drink a cup of schizandra decoction 2–3 times a day for a week using 25 g berries to 500 ml water.*
• *Damiana is a good aphrodisiac for men (take 1 ml of tincture in warm water 2–3 times daily), while chaste-tree berries work well on women (take 10 drops of tincture in warm water 3 times a day).*

EXHAUSTION

Long working hours, pregnancy, and a demanding family can exhaust even the fittest.

Remedies
• *Rest and relaxation are essential. Instead of caffeine, take Siberian ginseng capsules (2 x 200 mg up to 3 times daily) as a boost.*
• *Drink a tea made from equal amounts of dried vervain, rosemary, and gotu kola, 2–3 times a day. (Note: this quantity of vervain is safe in pregnancy, but do not exceed the dose or take for more than 2–3 weeks.)*

INDIGESTION

Stress and rushed mealtimes soon lead to indigestion with pain, gas, and heartburn. In pregnancy, the growing fetus often plays havoc with the digestion.

Remedies
• *Drink a cup of standard fennel or chamomile infusion after meals.*
• *To relieve heartburn and acidity, take 1–2 capsules filled with equal amounts of powdered slippery elm bark and marshmallow root.*
• *Chew crystallized ginger or drink peppermint infusion to relieve gas.*

PEPTIC ULCERS

This painful condition, caused by erratic meals and stress, is most common among those aged 30–40 years old. Ulcers require professional treatment, but the following remedies can relieve symptoms in controlled conditions.

Remedies
• *Make an infusion of 15 g each of dried meadowsweet and chamomile and take a cup up to 4 times daily.*
• *Take 1–2 capsules of 1 g slippery elm and 1 g San Qi 3 times daily.*

THE MIDDLE YEARS - MEN

— THE FIFTH LIFE STAGE —

SOME MEN experience an emotional midlife crisis as they see youth slipping away. This may result in a yearning for bygone days, or even lead to divorce and a search for a new, younger partner. Other men become depressed as they dwell on unfulfilled ambitions and the frustrations of failing strength. Fortunately the middle years are a very positive time for many men,

Linden flowers

encompassing wide interests and achievements, a comfortable lifestyle, and a happy family life, as children become less demanding and dependent. Such self-satisfaction brings its own problems: a tendency to eat too much and not get enough exercise. It is important to keep fit during the middle years as an investment for a healthy old age.

Preventative Treatments

Taking care to lead a healthy life is very important. Some of the following may also help guard against illness. For dosage advice on remedies, vitamins, and minerals, see p. 83. For instructions on making remedies, see pp. 62–79.

— HERBS —

LINDEN FLOWERS are ideal for stressed-out executives, encouraging relaxation and helping to reduce the risk of arteriosclerosis. Drink a cup of standard infusion regularly.

OATS are an excellent antidepressant and can also help reduce cholesterol levels. Eat oatmeal for breakfast or take 5 ml of oat tincture daily.

GARLIC reduces cholesterol levels and is strongly antibacterial, helping combat infections. Use plenty in cooking or take 2–3 garlic pearls daily.

— VITAMINS & MINERALS —

BETA-CAROTENE (vitamin A) has been identified by some as a valuable cancer preventative. Eat plenty of carrots or take up to 20,000 IUs daily.
Caution: Excessive vitamin A can be toxic.

VITAMIN E is helpful in combating coronary artery disease and poor circulation. Take 400 IUs daily.
Caution: Avoid, except under medical supervision, if taking blood-thinning drugs such as warfarin.

SELENIUM has been shown to help prevent cancer and reduce the risk of heart attacks. Take 100 µg daily.

TIMELY TONICS

DAMIANA
This is a stimulating, strengthening tonic which is reputedly an aphrodisiac. Take 1–2 cups of standard infusion daily.

Dried herb

KOREAN GINSENG
Korean, or Chinese, ginseng is a Yang tonic. Take 1–2 x 250 mg tablets or capsules a day. (Do not take if suffering from high blood pressure.)

Capsules

GOU QI ZI
These are associated with longevity and make a good liver and kidney tonic. Chew 2–3 berries or take a 200 mg capsule of the powdered herb daily.

Berries

BENZOIN
A good sedative, especially useful for urinary and respiratory problems. Add 5 drops to the bathwater or use in massage oils.

Oil

Health Profile

TOO MANY BUSINESS LUNCHES and no exercise can result in middle-aged spread. The middle years are also a time of severe illnesses, such as heart attacks, lung cancer, and digestive problems. Regular exercise and a healthy diet may help to prevent these problems.

HIGH BLOOD PRESSURE
Stress and weight gain increase the risk of high blood pressure and heart attacks. It is essential to seek professional help, but exercise, giving up smoking, relaxation, and careful weight control are all generally advised. The following remedies can help mild cases.

Remedies
- *Take a standard infusion daily made with equal parts dried hawthorn flowers, linden flowers, Ju Hua, and yarrow.*
- *Take 2.5 ml each of cramp bark and hawthorn berry tinctures 3 times a day.*

RHEUMATIC ACHES AND PAINS
The middle years are a time when some people are afflicted with joint pains. They are sometimes associated with developing arthritic disorders, and prompt treatment at this stage can prevent problems arising later on.

Remedies
- *Mix 2 ml rosemary oil, 1 ml lavender oil, and 2 ml thyme oil in 50 ml sweet almond oil. Massage gently into aching limbs.*
- *Take 2 x 200 mg devil's claw capsules 3 times a day.*
- *Mix 20 ml each of meadowsweet, celery seed, black cohosh, angelica root, and bogbean tinctures and take 5 ml 3 times a day.*

EYESTRAIN
In the middle years, the eyes become more farsighted, and many people need glasses. It is important to have an eye test regularly to check that glasses are the right strength.

Remedies
- *Add 5 drops of self-heal tincture to an eyewash of warm water and bathe the eyes.*
- *Apply used chamomile teabags to the eyes, lie down, and relax for 10 minutes.*
- *Drink a cup of Ju Hua standard infusion daily.*

PROSTATE PROBLEMS
Benign enlargement of the prostate gland is commonplace, leading to problems with urination. Seeking professional advice without delay is important, to eliminate the possibility of prostate cancer.

Remedies
- *Take 5 ml saw palmetto tincture in a little warm water 3 times a day, or take the herb in the form of over the-counter tablets (follow the dosage instructions on the pack).*
- *Drink a standard infusion of equal parts of damiana and white deadnettle 2–3 times daily.*

CIRCULATORY DISORDERS
Problems with circulation are frequently associated with smoking. Symptoms of poor circulation include cramplike leg pains and cold hands and feet.

Remedies
- *Try very hard to give up smoking.*
- *Circulatory stimulants such as prickly ash bark and cinnamon twigs can help: take 2 ml of either tincture 3 times daily in warm water.*
- *Drink a standard infusion of equal parts of dried linden and hawthorn 2–3 times a day.*

THE MIDDLE YEARS - WOMEN

THE FIFTH LIFE STAGE

FASHION DESIGNER Coco Chanel once said that women are born 18, 35, or 55 years old. For some, the middle years start early and middle-aged attitudes are adopted in their teens. Other women, however, retain their youthful exuberance to the end. The Chinese traditionally measured a woman's life in seven-year stretches, with menopause at 49 years marking an end to

Sage

reproductive and useful life. Today, no woman need regard the change of life in such negative terms. Glamorous role models in their middle fifties are commonplace, and although the departure of grown-up children can be traumatic and depressing for some mothers, the middle years are a time of freedom to discover new interests and activities.

Preventative Treatments

A good balanced diet should provide most nutrients, but the following treatments may be useful. For dosage advice on remedies, vitamins, and minerals, see p. 83. For instructions on making remedies, see pp. 62–79.

HERBS

SAGE, reputed to guarantee a long life, is also now known to mimic female hormones, making it a useful supplement during menopause. Drink a cup of standard infusion 1–2 times daily.

ST.-JOHN'S-WORT is restorative, antidepressant, ideal for fraught nerves and menopausal traumas. Take a cup of standard infusion daily.

VERVAIN is a calming nervine and liver tonic and some believe it has a spiritual action. Drink 1–2 cups of standard infusion daily.

VITAMINS & MINERALS

CALCIUM can help reduce the risk of osteoporosis in later life. Green vegetables, nuts, and legumes are good sources, or take a 1 g supplement daily.

MAGNESIUM is important for the metabolism of calcium. Leafy green vegetables are important dietary sources. Alternatively, take 400–800 mg daily.

VITAMIN E is an antioxidant and can be useful for reducing menopausal symptoms. Take 400 IUs daily. Caution: Avoid, except under medical supervision, if taking blood-thinning drugs such as warfarin.

TIMELY TONICS

DANG SHEN
The Chinese regard this as a good Yin tonic and a more gentle energy source than ginseng. Take a sherry glass of tonic wine or 2 x 200 mg capsules daily.

Tonic wine

NU ZHEN ZI
A liver and kidney tonic that is also traditionally taken to restore hair color. Take a sherry glass of tonic wine or 2 x 200 mg capsules daily.

Tonic wine

CHASTE-TREE BERRIES
These stimulate female hormones and can help regulate their production. Take 2 x 200 mg capsules or 2.5 ml tincture in warm water each day.

Capsules

CYPRESS OIL
The sedating and restraining effect of this oil can help with menopausal problems. Use in massage oils or add 5 drops to the bathwater.

Oil

Health Profile

FOR SOME, the middle years can be a time of menopausal problems and emotional upsets, with depression and loss of libido. But they can also be marked by new feelings of independence and self-confidence. A positive attitude to the change of life is essential. Regular exercise is important to maintain bone structure and guard against osteoporosis.

MENOPAUSAL SYNDROME

Menopausal women may experience hot flashes, night sweats, irregular or heavy periods, mood swings, and irritability. In traditional Chinese medicine these are linked with a reduction of kidney energy and are treated with tonic, restorative herbs.

Remedies

• *Night sweats can be reduced with sage and mugwort tea. Each evening, drink a large cup of standard infusion made with equal amounts of both herbs.*
• *Chaste-tree berries can help regulate erratic hormones. Take 2.5 ml tincture in a little warm water each morning.*
• *He Shou Wu is a good tonic. Try a sherry glass daily of tonic wine*

DRYNESS

Dry eyes and a dry vagina are common menopausal problems.

Remedies

• *To help dry eyes, drink a cup of standard infusion made with equal amounts of vervain, wood betony, and Ju Hua flowers.*
• *Vaginal dryness can be eased by using vitamin E or pot marigold creams. Apply a little morning and evening and before intercourse.*
• *Add 10–20 drops of chamomile oil or 500 ml infusion to bathwater. The infusion may also be used as a vaginal wash.*

ACNE ROSACEA

Starting with a persistent facial flush and progressing to acnelike pustules, this is particularly common during menopause. Alcohol, tea, and coffee make it worse and should be avoided.

Remedies

• *Use a lotion made with 50 ml pot marigold tincture, 50 ml rosewater, and 2 drops of rose oil. Apply to the rash 2–3 times a day.*

GALLBLADDER PROBLEMS

Gallstones and other gallbladder problems often occur in overweight, middle-aged women. The symptoms include acute colicky pain, and professional medical attention is required. Mild conditions may respond to simple home remedies.

Remedies

• *Try 2 ml each of fringe tree bark, fumitory, and vervain tinctures in warm water 3 times a day.*
• *To relieve symptoms, drink a cup every 2–3 hours of a standard decoction made with 15 g dandelion root, 10 g wild yam root, and 5 g barberry bark.*

DEPRESSION

The middle years can feel empty when children leave the nest and partners seem preoccupied with careers. Maintaining a strong image of self-worth is essential.

Remedies

• *Take 2 ml of vervain and oat tinctures with 1 ml of lemon balm tincture, in warm water 3 times daily.*
• *Drink a large cup 3–4 times daily of a standard infusion of equal parts St.-John's-wort and wood betony.*
• *Bach Flower Remedies can help. Try walnut to cope with change, and honeysuckle to stop the mind from dwelling on the past.*

THE NEWLY RETIRED

THE SIXTH LIFE STAGE

TODAY, RETIREMENT signals a new beginning: a chance to travel to exotic places or develop new interests and hobbies. Retirement however, is not always trouble-free: it is a time of major readjustment, that workaholics in particular often find difficult. Giving up the status and companionship that work brings, or living

Garlic bulb

on a reduced income, may lead to depression and lack of self-esteem in some people. Maintaining a positive attitude to life is essential. Recent research has associated both prostate problems and osteoporosis with a sedentary lifestyle, so gentle, enjoyable exercise, such as walking, bowling, golf, gardening, and cycling is important for both sexes.

Preventative Treatments

A healthy diet is perhaps one of the best investments for a healthy old age. In addition, the following can be useful.
For dosage advice on remedies, vitamins, and minerals, see p. 83. For instructions on making remedies, see pp. 62–79.

HERBS

GARLIC is especially valuable to help maintain health as old age approaches. Use plenty in cooking or take 2–3 pearls daily.

CINNAMON reduces blood sugar levels and is a useful tonic if the circulation is poor. Try powdered cinnamon sprinkled on hot buttered toast.

MOTHERWORT is a tonic herb for the heart and a gentle sedative. It also has a restorative effect on the female reproductive organs. Take a cup of standard infusion regularly.

VITAMINS & MINERALS

VITAMIN C, found in fresh fruit and vegetables, is important for everyone, but rheumatism sufferers in particular may benefit from taking a high dose (4 g daily) since it flushes out uric acid from the system and helps with gouty arthritis.

SELENIUM is an antioxidant, preventing cell damage. It is also thought to help maintain a healthy heart and muscles. Take 100–200 µg daily.

VITAMIN B$_1$ (thiamin) deficiency is linked to heart problems. Take 50 mg daily.

TIMELY TONICS

LING ZHI
Regarded by the Taoists as a tonic for long life, this is ideal at times of change to help resolve the will. Take 2 x 200 mg capsules or 10 ml tincture daily.

Tincture

KOREAN GINSENG
The ideal tonic for the older person. Take 1–2 x 250 mg tablets or capsules or 10 ml tincture daily. Avoid prolonged use if suffering from high blood pressure.

Tincture

BASIL
In India this herb is regarded as a potent spiritual tonic, encouraging faith, compassion, and clarity. Take 5 ml of juice daily.

Juice

DANG SHEN
An energy tonic that can be particularly helpful for women and also eases tension. Take a sherry glass of tonic wine or 2 x 200 mg capsules daily.

Capsules

Health Profile

As the body ages, the frustration of aching limbs, lack of stamina, insomnia, or failing eyesight can be daunting. Accepting that physical energies are gradually slowing down, staying as healthy as possible, and making the most of every day are important lessons. This life stage is a time when any physical abuse will come home to roost: decades of poor diet can lead to late-onset diabetes, for example, and habitual use of laxatives may result in diverticulitis.

ANGINA PECTORIS

Angina, related to disease of the coronary arteries, is characterized by sharp pains in the chest, arms, shoulders, or neck. Professional treatment is essential but can be augmented with medicinal herbs.

Remedies
* If high cholesterol levels are a contributory factor, take 4 x 200 mg garlic capsules or 2 cloves daily.
* Drink a standard infusion of equal parts of hawthorn, motherwort, and linden flowers 3 times a day.
* Take 10 drops of San Qi tincture in water 3 times a day.

LUMBAGO & SCIATICA

Sciatic pain may run from lower back to the knee and is exacerbated by excessive gardening. Lumbago is a term for pain in the lower back.

Remedies
* Add 5 drops each of pine, geranium, and peppermint oils to an evening bath and enjoy a long soak. Mix the same oils in 10 ml of infused St.-John's-wort oil and gently massage the affected areas.

ARTHRITIS

Osteoarthritis is caused by general wear-and-tear on the joints and can very quickly limit activity as joints stiffen and pain becomes a misery.

Remedies
* Take 2 x 200 mg capsules of devil's claw 3 times a day for at least 4 weeks.
* Massage infused comfrey oil or comfrey cream into the affected joint twice a day. Continue for at least 2 months.

LATE-ONSET DIABETES

A tendency to develop this condition can be hereditary. It can also be caused by obesity, and a lifetime of high sugar consumption. Early symptoms include fatigue, excessive thirst, and increased urination. Professional help is vital.

Remedies
* Take 2 x 200 mg capsules of fenugreek 3 times a day before meals.
* Drink a cup of standard infusion of equal parts goat's rue and bilberry leaves 3 times a day.
* Use plenty of garlic in cooking, or take 2–3 pearls daily.

DIVERTICULITIS

Excessive use of laxatives and low-fiber diets can weaken the bowel wall, and create small pouches (diverticuli), which become inflamed and infected by trapped food particles.

Remedies
* Drink a cup 3 times daily of standard decoction of wild yam and marshmallow root, flavored with a little licorice extract.
* Drink a cup of standard chamomile infusion regularly to help reduce inflammation.

THE ELDERLY

THE SEVENTH LIFE STAGE

A CENTURY AGO, most people in the West thought those over 50 were elderly. Today, the number of over-70s in our society continues to grow steadily and many more people live to 80 or 90 years of age. But no matter how vigorous the individual is, the ills of old age catch up eventually. Despite the skills of modern medicine, cancer and cardiovascular disease

Stinging nettle

remain the developed world's greatest scourges, and the risk of suffering from either inevitably increases with age. A varied diet with lots of fresh fruit and vegetables is now recognized as a preventative factor for both diseases. Unfortunately, apathy often leads to missed meals, so this is a life stage when vitamin and mineral supplements are particularly valuable.

Preventative Treatments

Taking care to follow a healthy lifestyle is very important and the following herbs, vitamins, and minerals can further boost health. For dosage advice on remedies, vitamins, and minerals, see p. 83. For instructions on making remedies, see pp. 62–79.

HERBS

STINGING NETTLES are rich in minerals and vitamins and can supplement a deficient diet. Drink a cup of standard infusion daily.

GOTU KOLA is a good nerve tonic used in Ayurvedic medicine to encourage mental calm and clarity. Drink a cup of standard infusion regularly.

KELP, OR BLADDERWRACK, is rich in iodine and other minerals and is a gentle metabolic stimulant. It is very helpful in debility. Take 3–6 x 400 mg tablets daily.

VITAMINS & MINERALS

B VITAMINS deficiency can lead to cracked corners of the mouth and a sore, red tongue. Take 1–2 g tablets of a good quality B-complex supplement daily.

VITAMIN C is important to combat infection and many progressive diseases. Eat plenty of fresh fruit and vegetables or take 1–2 g supplement daily.

COD LIVER OIL reduces the risk of heart disease. Use combined fish and evening primrose oil capsules (take 500–750 mg daily).

TIMELY TONICS

AMERICAN GINSENG
This has a more Yin character than Korean ginseng and can be more suitable for the very elderly. Take 1–2 x 250 mg tablets daily or a sherry glass of tonic wine.

Tonic wine

OATS
Oats are an excellent tonic food, antidepressant, and restorative. Make oatmeal from freshly milled oats and eat regularly.

Oatmeal

SAGE
This herb is traditionally associated in the West with longevity. Drink a cup of standard infusion every day.

Dried herb

GINKGO BILOBA
This herb is known to encourage the circulation of blood to the brain and reduces confusion in the elderly. Take 3 x 200 mg tablets or 10 ml tincture daily.

Tablets

Health Profile

OLD AGE BRINGS its fair share of health problems as energies wane and parts of the body show signs of wear and tear. Fatigue, insomnia, and poor appetite are common, and general weakness can lead to problems with the digestion, urinary system, and circulation. It is important to keep warm and stay as active as possible, and it is also wise to maintain contacts with people of all ages and retain a lively interest in current events.

HEARING PROBLEMS
Deafness and tinnitus limit normal conversation and add to isolation. White-noise cassette tapes can ease severe tinnitus, and herbs can prove surprisingly helpful.

Remedies
• *Combine 25 ml each of tinctures of* ginkgo biloba, *pasque flower,* Nu Zhen Zi, *and schizandra berries and take 50 drops in water 3 times daily.*
• *Take a 200 mg capsule of goldenseal 3 times a day if phlegm is a contributory problem.*

CONFUSION AND FORGETFULNESS
With age, short-term memory can become impaired. Senile dementia is common and needs understanding and patience from the family as well as professional medical support.

Remedies
• *Drink a standard infusion daily of dried gingko leaves and wood betony to improve circulation to the brain.*
• *Rosemary, and basil oils are gentle mental stimulants. Add 5 drops of each to the bathwater.*

CONSTIPATION
Constipation in the elderly can often be caused by general weakness of the digestive system as well as poor diet. Eat plenty of fiber but avoid too much bran, which can be an irritant.

Remedies
• *The Chinese used* Huo Ma Ren *(cannabis seeds) for constipation in the elderly. Sterile seeds are sold by specialist suppliers: make a decoction and drink a cup 3 times a day.*
• *Take 2.5 ml of* Dang Gui *tincture in half a glass of warm water 3 times a day.*

INCONTINENCE
Stress incontinence is common in women who have had children and it affects both sexes in old age. The following herbal remedies can be useful.

Remedies
• *Add 10 drops of cypress oil to 5 ml of sweet almond oil. Massage into the lower abdomen 2–3 times a day.*
• *Take 10 ml of horsetail juice twice a day.*
• *Take a standard decoction of equal amounts of* Huang Qi, Dang Gui, *and* Chi Shao Yao *3 times a day to alleviate symptoms.*

BRITTLE BONES
Hip fractures are a hazard and severe osteoporosis can lead to a curved spine. Regular exercise and plenty of magnesium and calcium are good preventative measures.

Remedies
• *Sage tea contains estrogen like substances that may help prevent loss of calcium from bones. Take a cup of standard infusion daily.*
• *Take a heaping teaspoon of freshly crushed linseed daily.*

A-to-Z of

MEDICINAL HERBS

OF THE MANY HUNDREDS of medicinal herbs available, the 60 in this index represent some of the most versatile and readily available, commonly used in both home remedies and over-the-counter preparations. These herbs feature frequently in the *Remedies for Common Ailments* section (pp. 82–137) and detailed instructions are given there on how to use them. All the herbs listed are safe for home use, although in some cases there are significant cautions that should be noted.

Achillea millefolium
YARROW

Yarrow was once known as "nosebleed," its feathery leaves making an ideal astringent swab to encourage clotting. It is an important herb for treating wounds, taking its name from the Greek hero, Achilles, who used it for just that. The plant was also important in fortune-telling, and yarrow stalks are still used by the Chinese for casting *I Ching* predictions.

Fresh aerial parts

Essential oil

Fresh leaves

PARTS USED: Aerial parts, essential oil.

KEY USES: Although useful as a wound herb, yarrow is mostly used for fevers and to relax blood vessels in high blood pressure. It is a bitter tasting digestive tonic, and is added to remedies to relieve menstrual and urinary disorders.

CAUTIONS:
• Can cause skin rashes.
• Use with caution during pregnancy.

Agrimonia eupatoria
AGRIMONY

Agrimony is found growing in hedge-rows, its tall yellow summer flowers giving it the folk name of "church steeples." It is a member of the rose family and, like all its relatives, is highly astringent. Indeed, it is a valuable wound herb, and was once a much-used remedy on medieval battlefields.

Fresh aerial parts

Dried aerial parts

PARTS USED: Aerial parts.

KEY USES: Like many astringent herbs, agrimony can be helpful for diarrhea, and it is especially suitable for children. It can effectively stop bleeding from cuts and scrapes, and taken internally, can ease heavy menstrual bleeding and acute, severe cystitis.

Allium sativum
GARLIC

The Ancient Egyptians spoke of garlic as a potent remedy for coughs and colds – for which it is still prized today. In many countries garlic is the most popular over-the-counter herbal remedy. Its potent chemicals can only be excreted through the lungs and skin, hence the aromatic consequences of high doses.

Fresh bulb

Fresh cloves

PARTS USED: Cloves.

KEY USES: Garlic is antiseptic and antifungal. It also helps reduce blood cholesterol levels.

CAUTION:
• Excessive topical use may cause irritation.

Althaea officinalis
MARSHMALLOW

The Romans looked on marshmallow as a culinary delight and the sweet, juicy roots are said to be quite palatable if fried with onions and butter. Medicinally, its mucilaginous (soft, slippery) nature makes marshmallow ideal for soothing respiratory and digestive disorders. It is a very pretty plant – well worth growing in a damp corner of the garden.

PARTS USED: Leaves, root, flowers.

KEY USES: Marshmallow is used as an expectorant for chest coughs and bronchitis. It is also very soothing for inflamed mucous membranes, especially in the digestive tract and urinary system.

Fresh flowers

Anemone vulgaris
PASQUE FLOWER

Pasque flower is so called because its purple flowers were once used to stain eggshells red at Easter. It is a popular garden plant, and used medicinally is a very effective sedative, especially for painful conditions.

PARTS USED: Aerial parts, dried (the fresh plant is toxic.)

KEY USES: Pasque flower is especially effective for menstrual pain and other painful conditions of the reproductive system in both men and women. It also seems to act well in urinary disorders and, when taken internally, can relieve earache.

CAUTIONS:
• Do not exceed stated dose.
• Do not use the fresh plant.

Flowering plant

Dried aerial parts

Fresh plant

Fresh root

Angelica sinensis
DANG GUI/ CHINESE ANGELICA

Dang Gui is one of China's most popular tonic herbs and is now being used in many Western patent remedies as well. It is particularly suitable for women, and has been taken for thousands of years as a restorative after childbirth to fortify blood in anemic conditions and to beautify the skin.

Dried root

PARTS USED: Root.

KEY USES: *Dang Gui* acts on the female reproductive system, is a good liver remedy, circulatory stimulant and blood tonic.

CAUTION:
• Avoid in pregnancy.

Dried leaves

Apium graveolens
CELERY

Thanks to modern agriculture, celery has now become an all-year-round vegetable. At one time, however, it was only ready for cutting in winter and spring, when it was used as a effective cleansing herbal tonic at a time when little fresh food was available. The seeds are used medicinally.

PARTS USED: Seeds.

KEY USES: Celery seed is a diuretic, and is the best remedy for clearing uric acid from the system. It is ideal for gout, arthritis and rheumatism. It can also be useful to treat cystitis and related problems.

CAUTIONS:
• Only use seeds sold for medicinal purposes, as those intended for planting are often treated with fungicide.
• Avoid high doses in pregnancy as it can cause abortion.

Fresh stalk

Dried seeds

Arctium lappa
BURDOCK

Burdock and dandelion cordial can still be found in stores. It is a reminder of what was once a popular spring-cleaning combination, combating constipation and stagnation disorders.

PARTS USED: Leaves, root, seeds.

KEY USES: Burdock is a good cleansing herb for arthritis and various skin conditions, and it is also a digestive stimulant and mild laxative. The root is mostly used although the leaves have a similar, gentler action. The Chinese use the seeds as a remedy for feverish colds.

CAUTION:
• The growing plant may cause contact dermatitis.

Dried leaves

Dried seeds

Fresh plant

Dried root

Arnica montana
ARNICA

Arnica is a daisy-like plant, found in rich, peaty, alpine pastures. Taken internally it can be extremely toxic, so it is only used in homeopathic preparations, which are very dilute. In the form of creams and ointments, however, it is one of the most useful in the herbal repertoire.

Fresh flowers

Fresh plant

PARTS USED: Flowers.

KEY USES: Arnica cream can be used for conditions where poor circulation is a contributory factor, such as frostbite, or where the circulatory system needs some stimulation to encourage healing. Arnica ointment and an internal arnica homeopathic remedy are a good combination for traumatic shocks or accidents.

CAUTIONS:
• Do not use the cream on broken skin.
• Only take homeopathic doses internally.

Astragalus membranaceus
HUANG QI/ ASTRAGALUS

Huang Qi has been used as an energy tonic by the Chinese for thousands of years, although more recent interest in the herb focuses on its immune-stimulating properties. The plant, known in English as "milk vetch," is a member of the bean family and can be grown in temperate areas.

Dried root

PARTS USED: Root.

KEY USES: The Chinese look on *Huang Qi* as a young person's tonic. It is ideal for conditions related to immune deficiency, such as when repeated colds or allergies weaken natural resistance. It is becoming more widely used in Western over-the-counter remedies.

Barosma betulina
BUCHU

This tall, South African shrub has a characteristic blackcurrant flavor, making it one of the more palatable medicinal herbs. It originates from Cape Province and was originally used by local Hottentot tribes, both medicinally and in body perfumes.

PARTS USED: Leaves.

Dried leaves

KEY USES: Buchu is an effective urinary antiseptic, ideal for cystitis and similar conditions. It is a warming and stimulating herb and makes a useful kidney tonic.

Calendula officinalis
POT MARIGOLD

In the 17th century, pot marigold was regarded as an ideal cure for "plague and pestilence," a more effective remedy than other plague potions as marigold is highly antiseptic. Its bright orange flowers were also supposed to strengthen the heart, while simply looking at these cheerful plants was recommended to lift the spirits.

Fresh plant

PARTS USED: Petals.

KEY USES: Marigold, commonly available as a cream, makes a useful antiseptic, antifungal and astringent remedy for many skin problems, inflammations and minor injuries. Taken internally, it is an effective bile stimulant, useful for the digestive system, and it can also ease menstrual problems.

Dried petals

Capsella bursa-pastoris
SHEPHERD'S PURSE

This common, garden weed has been used medicinally worldwide for at least 2,000 years. In the 17th century, sprigs of it, bound to the hands and feet, were recommended for jaundice, while ointments made from the herb were used on wounds. It is also known as "mother's hearts" because of the shape of its seed pods.

Dried aerial parts

PARTS USED: Aerial parts.

KEY USES: A useful herb to stop external and internal bleeding, it is used mainly to treat urinary and menstrual disorders. It is also a circulatory stimulant and is useful as a wound remedy.

CAUTION:
• Avoid in pregnancy, although it can be helpful during labor.

Fresh aerial parts

Capsicum frutescens
CHILI/CAYENNE

Chili peppers arrived in Europe from India in the 16th century and were initially used for virulent skin conditions. The herbalist John Gerard disliked the plant, saying that it would "kill dogs." Chilies are, of course, extremely hot and need to be used with caution.

Fresh fruits

Oil

Ointment

PARTS USED: Fruit.

KEY USES: Chilies are warming and stimulating, and can be taken in remedies for colds, chills, rheumatic pains, poor circulation, and nervous shocks. Ointments and oils help to stimulate blood flow to an area, or to ease the lingering pain from a shingles attack.

CAUTIONS:
• Do not take the seeds – they can be toxic.
• Avoid touching the eyes or cuts after handling fresh chilies.
• External use may cause dermatitis.

Cimicifuga racemosa
BLACK COHOSH

Black cohosh was used by various Native American tribes for rheumatism, kidney problems, exhaustion, and gynecological disorders. The herb was listed in the US *Pharmacopeia* from 1820 to 1936. It is a member of the buttercup family, with cream flower spikes and a distinctive black root.

Fresh root

PARTS USED: Root.

KEY USES: Black cohosh is a useful remedy for all sorts of muscle pains and cramps. It is an effective muscle relaxant for spasmodic conditions, including menstrual cramps, and also appears to have some hormonal actions.

CAUTIONS:
• Do not exceed the stated dose.
• Avoid in pregnancy.

Cinnamomum zeylanicum
CINNAMON

In Roman times, cinnamon was reputed to grow only in remote marshes protected by monstrous bats, a tale that Pliny suggested was circulated by the spice merchants to keep the price high. The bark has been exported from Sri Lanka and India for more than 2,000 years.

Dried bark

Sticks of bark

Powdered bark

Dried twigs

PARTS USED: Bark, twigs, essential oil.

KEY USES: Cinnamon bark is a warming digestive remedy. It also has a tonic effect on the kidneys, helps stimulate the circulation, and makes an effective tea for common colds. The essential oil can be used in chest rubs or abdominal massage for colic.

Citrus aurantium
BITTER ORANGE

Bitter oranges are most familiar these days in traditional English marmalade, although the essential oils (neroli distilled from the flowers and bergamot from the fruit) are also well known. The Chinese use both the ripe and immature fruits in medicine.

Fresh fruit

Neroli oil

Zhi Ke (ripe fruit)

Zhi Shi (unripe fruit)

PARTS USED: Fruit, peel, essential oils.

KEY USES: Bitter oranges are carminative for gas and indigestion, and can also relieve nausea. Both neroli and bergamot oils are widely used in aromatherapy, acting on the nervous and digestive systems.

Dioscorea villosa
WILD YAM

The wild yam was the original starting point for making the first oral contraceptives – thanks to the hormonal compound, diosgenin, it contains. The Aztecs regarded it as a relaxing digestive remedy, which is how herbalists still use it today.

Dried root

PARTS USED: Root.

KEY USES: Wild yam is a good anti-spasmodic for the digestive and reproductive system, especially helpful for irritable bowel syndrome or for menstrual pain.

CAUTION:
• Avoid in pregnancy, although it may be taken during labor.

Echinacea angustifolia
ECHINACEA

The Native Americans used echinacea, also known as "purple coneflower," for snakebites, fevers, and wounds. The herb soon became popular with the early settlers; today it is appreciated as an important immune stimulant and antibacterial, ideal for almost any sort of infection.

PARTS USED: Root.

KEY USES: Whenever there is infection – viral, bacterial, or fungal – echinacea has a role. It is the ideal choice for colds, flu, and kidney infections and can be helpful in viral-based arthritis and for sore throats. It can also be applied externally for some skin conditions.

Dried root

Fresh flower

Fresh root

Eleutherococcus senticosus
SIBERIAN GINSENG

Siberian ginseng is a relative newcomer to the herbal repertoire. Only widely used since the 1930s, it is ideal for combating the stresses of 20th-century life. It was once a favorite with both Soviet athletes and long distance truck drivers, who took it regularly to increase stamina and improve performance.

Dried root

PARTS USED: Root.

KEY USES: Ideal whenever stress is proving a problem, Siberian ginseng is a useful herb to take before exams or a busy time at work. It can also be helpful as a remedy for nervous exhaustion and lack of energy.

Eschscholzia californica
CALIFORNIA POPPY

The California poppy is a common garden flower. Known as "nightcap" in the US, it is a gentle and very useful sedative, ideal for sleeplessness, even in children. Unlike some members of the poppy family, it has no addictive side-effects and is quite safe to use.

PARTS USED: Aerial parts.

KEY USES: A gentle sedative for the nervous system, this herb is excellent for insomnia, stress or tension, and can be pleasantly taken in teas at any time. It can also be very helpful for overactive digestive systems.

Fresh aerial parts

Eucalyptus globulus
EUCALYPTUS

Once a favorite cure-all for the Australian Aborigines, eucalyptus is mainly used today for infections and chest problems. Current research suggests it is a very potent antibacterial. The tree grows well in temperate climates although it is tropical in origin.

Fresh leaves

PARTS USED: Essential oil.

KEY USES: Eucalyptus is best used as an external remedy. The oil is ideal in chest rubs and inhalants to treat all sorts of respiratory problems, and, used in massage oils, it is warming and soothing for rheumatic aches and pains.

Essential oil

Euphrasia officinalis
EYEBRIGHT

Eyebright is a nondescript, semiparasitic plant found mainly in meadows and chalk downland, yet it is one of the most effective antiphlegm remedies. As its name suggests, it is also used as an eye remedy, and, indeed, was a favorite with great 17th-century herbalists such as Nicholas Culpeper.

Fresh aerial parts

PARTS USED: Aerial parts.

KEY USES: Eyebright relieves congestion and phlegm, and is useful in remedies for hay fever and common colds. It can be taken internally or used in eye baths as a soothing remedy for many eye infections and irritations.

Filipendula ulmaria
MEADOWSWEET

In the 1830s anti-inflammatory chemicals were first extracted from meadowsweet, and in the 1890s the world's first patent drug appeared, as "aspirin," taking its name from the old Latin name for meadowsweet, *Spiraea ulmaria*. The herb has always been a favorite for fevers and rheumatic pains, but unlike modern aspirin, it does not irritate the stomach lining.

PARTS USED: Aerial parts.

KEY USES: A good soothing remedy for the stomach, it is helpful for gastritis, stomach upsets, and many other digestive problems. Meadowsweet is also an excellent anti-inflammatory for arthritis and rheumatic conditions.

CAUTION:
• Meadowsweet is rich in salicylates, avoid in cases of aspirin allergy.

Foeniculum officinalis
FENNEL

The Ancient Greeks called fennel *marathron*, a word believed to mean "to grow thin," and used it as a dieting aid. Medieval churchgoers used to chew the seeds during boring sermons to stop stomach rumbles. Today, Florence fennel is a popular garden vegetable, useful in salads, while the original herb is still important for digestive remedies.

PARTS USED: Seeds.

KEY USES: A useful herb for digestive problems, it is ideal for indigestion, nausea, or to relieve griping pains. Fennel is also used to encourage milk flow in nursing mothers and can be taken to help respiratory complaints.

Fresh plant

Seeds

Glycyrrhiza glabra
LICORICE

For more than 2,500 years licorice has been used in medicine, both in Western Europe and in the Far East. The Chinese call it "the grandfather of herbs" and use it in many prescriptions to help balance other ingredients. It is also used to flavor many medicines. Licorice is a member of the bean family and grows well in temperate climates.

Fresh root

Fresh leaves

Dried root

Galium aparine
CLEAVERS

One of the most common weeds, cleavers is also known as "goosegrass" (because geese like to eat it) and "sweetheart" (for the way it clings to shrubs.) It has an ancient reputation as a spring tonic, traditionally taken as a cleansing remedy after the long winter.

PARTS USED: Aerial parts.

KEY USES: A good cleansing herb and lymphatic tonic, it is useful in many skin disorders and also for glandular problems, including tonsillitis and glandular fever.

Fresh aerial parts

Dried aerial parts

Fresh aerial parts

Dried aerial parts

PARTS USED: Root.

KEY USES: Licorice is a soothing digestive remedy, helpful for both gastric ulceration and diarrhea. It is also an expectorant and helpful for problem coughs such as in bronchitis and asthma. The herb encourages the production of many hormones, such as hydrocortisone, an anti-inflammatory.

CAUTIONS:
• Avoid excessive use in cases of high blood pressure, or other heart disease.
• Licorice should not be taken by people on digoxin-based drugs.

Hydrastis canadensis
GOLDENSEAL

One of the most popular digestive remedies among Native American tribes, goldenseal became a favorite with 19th-century herbalists both in America and Europe. The pioneers used to chew it for sore mouths and stomach upsets, although its bitterness would deter most modern sufferers. Goldenseal belongs to the buttercup family and only grows in a warm climate.

Fresh root

PARTS USED: Root.

KEY USES: A good antiphlegm remedy and liver stimulant, goldenseal is useful for many respiratory, digestive and menstrual problems, and can also be used externally for some skin conditions.

CAUTION:
• Avoid in pregnancy and in cases of high blood pressure.

Hypericum perforatum
ST.-JOHN'S-WORT

St.-John's-wort was once hung above doorways during midsummer to ward off evil spirits, and the red extract produced from its flowerheads was believed to be ideal for treating wounds and inflammations. Some say its name derives from the Knights of St. John of Jerusalem, who used it to heal wounds during the Crusades.

PARTS USED: Aerial parts, flowering tops.

KEY USES: St.-John's-wort is a good external anti-inflammatory, suitable for burns, wounds, and joint problems. It is also used for nervous disorders including depression and anxiety. In recent years, extracts have been tested for alleviating immune-deficiency problems.

CAUTION:
• Prolonged use can lead to photosensitivity.

Hyssopus officinalis
HYSSOP

Hyssop was used as a cure for asthma and catarrh by the Ancient Greeks, although the plant known from the Bible ["purge me with hyssop and I shall be clean" (*Psalm* 51)] is now believed to be a variety of marjoram. In the past it was also used for treating some forms of epilepsy. It forms an attractive, shrubby plant, useful in the garden to repel cabbage white butterflies.

PARTS USED: Aerial parts, essential oil.

KEY USES: Hyssop is a valuable respiratory remedy, and is especially good for children. It is a bitter stimulant that can be taken for digestive disorders.

Fresh aerial parts

Essential oil

Dried aerial parts

Fresh aerial parts

Fresh flower

Dried aerial parts

Juniperus communis
JUNIPER

Juniper has long been associated with ritual purifications and its smoke is still used to purge Eastern temples. It was also used in Ancient Egypt for mummification. Today, the herb is mainly regarded as an important urinary antiseptic, while the essential oils are used for arthritis and psoriasis.

PARTS USED: Berries, essential oils.

KEY USES: The herb is taken internally to alleviate cystitis and urinary infections. Oil from the berries is used for chest problems and aches and pains, while oil from the twigs is useful for skin conditions.

CAUTIONS:
• Do not use in pregnancy.
• Avoid using for more than 6 weeks as the herb can irritate the mucous membranes.

Lactuca virosa
WILD LETTUCE

Beatrix Potter's bunnies fell asleep after eating too much lettuce – a good example of this herb's sedative properties! Until the 1930s, extracts of the sap were sold as "lettuce opium," which was recommended as a painkiller and a treatment for insomnia and anxiety. The herb is most potent as it goes to seed; cultivated lettuce leaves used in salad have little potency.

Fresh aerial parts

PARTS USED: Aerial parts.

KEY USES: A sedative for anxiety, and other nervous problems, the herb can also soothe coughs, relax overactive digestive systems, and relieve muscular pains.

CAUTION:
• Do not exceed the stated dose; over-dosage is extremely toxic.
• The fresh plant may irritate the skin.

Fresh berries on stem

Essential oil

Lavandula officinalis
LAVENDER

Lavender is a favorite in herb gardens, where it is prized for its delightful scent. The Romans used it to scent bath water, hence its name, which comes from the Latin verb to wash (*lavare*). It was pre-scribed for coughs by the Ancient Greeks.

Fresh flowers

Essential oil

PARTS USED: Flowers, essential oil.

KEY USES: Lavender is generally regarded as an effective sedative and calming remedy for the digestion. It is ideal for migraines and headaches, either taken internally or used externally as a massage oil. Lavender oil is also soothing for sunburn, and makes a relaxing and uplifting addition to baths.

CAUTION:
• Avoid high doses in pregnancy.

Lonicera japonica
HONEYSUCKLE

The Chinese have long used honeysuckle flowers (*Jin Yin Hua*) as a cooling remedy for feverish colds, while in the West they have been recommended for chest problems and urinary infections since Roman times. In 17th-century England, Nicholas Culpeper considered "honeysuckle conserve" an essential ingredient for the household dispensary.

PARTS USED: Flowers.

KEY USES: Both the traditional European variety (*L. periclymenum*) and the more familiar Chinese plant can be used for chest colds and coughs. Honeysuckle is also useful for feverish conditions, including the aches and pains of flu and other inflammations.

Fresh buds

Dried buds

Fresh plant

Matricaria recutita
CHAMOMILE

The Anglo-Saxons looked on chamomile or "maythen" as one of the nine sacred herbs given to heal the world by the god Woden. The plant has a very distinctive smell – described by the Ancient Greeks as "ground apple," and produces pungent flowers for homemade chamomile tea.

PARTS USED: Flowers, essential oil.

KEY USES: A good sedative and calming herb for the digestive system, chamomile is also a favorite for babies and children, easing colic and teething pains. It is good for insomnia, and is also valuable for skin conditions and irritations.

CAUTIONS:
• Do not use chamomile oil in pregnancy.
• The fresh, growing plant may cause a contact skin rash in sensitive individuals.

Fresh plant

Melaleuca alternifolia
TEA TREE

The healing attributes of oil from the Australian tea tree were first investigated by the French in the 1920s and it has proved to be one of the most popular herbal antiseptics. Today it is widely used in many commercial preparations, and is important as an antifungal and antibacterial in many infectious conditions.

Fresh plant

PARTS USED: Essential oil.

KEY USES: It is used as an antiseptic for many skin infections such as thrush and acne. The oil can also be used in chest rubs or inhalants for colds and makes a useful hair rinse for head lice.

Essential oil

Melilotus officinalis
MELILOT

Also known as "king's clover," melilot is a striking, yellow field plant, which gives off a characteristic smell of new-mown hay as it dries. It was once the main ingredient of a favorite all-purpose household ointment, and today it is still used for treating skin conditions as well as vein problems.

PARTS USED: Aerial parts.

Fresh aerial parts

KEY USES: The herb helps to repair damage to blood vessels so it can be helpful for varicose veins or in creams for varicose eczema. Melilot is also used for some types of menstrual pain, depression, and insomnia, and is especially suitable for the elderly.

CAUTION:
• Melilot should not be taken by people on anticlotting drugs such as warfarin.

Dried leaves

Melissa officinalis
LEMON BALM

Lemon balm was used in 18th-century elixirs reputed to give everlasting youth, and was believed to "chase away melancholy." It is still used today as an antidepressant and is a valuable digestive herb. It is easy to grow, but it is an enthusiastic self-seeder and can become a nuisance in small gardens.

Fresh leaves

PARTS USED: Leaves, essential oil.

KEY USES: Taken internally, lemon balm is valuable for digestive upsets and nervous problems. The essential oil can be used in creams for wounds and for insect bites while its strong lemon scent also helps to keep mosquitoes away when used as a body rub.

Dried leaves

Essential oil

Oenothera biennis
EVENING PRIMROSE

Evening primrose oil has become one of the most popular over-the-counter supplements in recent years, due to its high gamma-linolenic acid content. This essential fatty acid is vital to maintain normal bodily functions, although fortunately, most people can make it themselves internally. The distinctive yellow flowers of evening primrose are common on waste-ground in the summer.

PARTS USED: Seed oil.

KEY USES: The extracted seed oil is used for a very wide range of conditions, including skin problems, menstrual irregularities, arthritis, and alcohol abuse.

Fresh plant

Seed oil

Mentha piperita
PEPPERMINT

Mints readily cross-breed and peppermint is a cross between watermint and spearmint, or garden mint. It has been well established in Europe for at least 1,000 years. It is used to flavor liqueurs, such as Chartreuse and Crème de Menthe, and is widely cultivated for its oil.

PARTS USED: Aerial parts, essential oil.

KEY USES: A good digestive remedy, peppermint oil can also be helpful for respiratory problems and skin complaints. The herb is ideal in cold remedies, for aches and pains and for some types of headaches and migraine.

CAUTIONS:
• The essential oil can be an irritant. Avoid prolonged use and do not give to young babies.
• Peppermint can reduce milk flow during breast-feeding.

Fresh aerial parts

Essential oil

Dried aerial parts

Panax ginseng
GINSENG

Ginseng has been known in the West since the days of Marco Polo, although its widespread use dates only from the 18th century. The Chinese have used the root (*Ren Shen*) of this plant as an energy tonic for at least 5,000 years, and today it forms the basis of many patent remedies. Most roots are now commercially cultivated, as wild plants are scarce.

Fresh root

PARTS USED: Root.

KEY USES: This strong energy tonic has been popular with elderly Chinese for centuries. It is also a good lung remedy and can help to speed recovery in chronic chest conditions.

CAUTIONS:
• Avoid high doses or prolonged use in pregnancy.
• If taking ginseng regularly, it is best to take a short break from the herb every couple of months, and limit other herbal stimulants and caffeine.

Petroselinum crispum
PARSLEY

Like nettles, parsley robs the soil of many minerals and vitamins and concentrates them in its leaves, making this traditional garnish a healthy part of a meal. The Ancient Greeks associated the plant with death and glory, and used it as fodder for their warhorses and decoration for their tombs. It does not like being transplanted, so is best sown where it will grow.

Fresh plant

PARTS USED: Leaves.

KEY USES: A good diuretic and dietary supplement, parsley can be helpful for many urinary problems as well as fluid retention associated with menstrual irregularities. Its concentrated minerals make it a valuable supplement for anemia. It also encourages milk flow in nursing mothers.

CAUTION:
• High consumption of the leaf is best avoided in pregnancy.

Plantago spp.
PLANTAIN

Once known as "waybread," common plantain (*P. major*) was one of the Anglo-Saxons' sacred herbs. The Native Americans called it "white man's foot" because it followed the settlers. Both common plantain and the taller ribwort species (*P. lanceolata*) are used medicinally; common plantain is used as a first aid remedy for bee stings, while ribwort plantain is important as a digestive and respiratory remedy for a range of phlegm-associated conditions.

Fresh leaf
(P. lanceolata)

Dried leaves (P. lanceolata)

PARTS USED: Leaves.

KEY USES: Ribwort plantain is a good antiphlegm remedy for colds and allergic rhinitis. It is also a soothing digestive remedy for various types of gastric irritation and inflammation and makes a useful external poultice for stings and slow-healing wounds.

Polygonum multiflorum
HE SHOU WU/ FO TI

He Shou Wu (known as *Fo Ti* in the US) is one of the most important Chinese tonic herbs and is believed by the Taoists to bring longevity and wisdom. It was traditionally drunk daily as a tonic wine and was reputed to dispel grey hairs and increase reproductive energy. Its English name is "fleeceflower."

Dried root

PARTS USED: Root.

KEY USES: As a tonic herb, *He Shou Wu* can be especially helpful for menopausal women. It is believed by the Chinese to boost creative energy, so it is useful for hard-working executives suffering from creativity "burn-out." In China it is also given for some heart disorders and is used externally for sores.

CAUTION:
• Only the prepared variety, obtainable from Chinese herb shops, should be used.

Fresh leaf
(P. major)

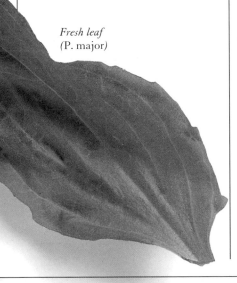

Rosmarinus officinalis
ROSEMARY

Rosemary has long been regarded in Europe as a stimulating herb that helps to dispel melancholy. According to Gerard in the 16th century it "maketh the harte merrie." The herb traditionally signified remembrance and was exchanged by lovers or left on tombs. Its stimulant properties are due to chemicals in the aromatic oil, which is extracted and used in aromatherapy.

Fresh aerial parts

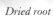

Essential oil

Dried aerial parts

PARTS USED: Aerial parts, essential oil.

KEY USES: The herb is a good digestive tonic and a carminative. It also helps stimulate the nervous system, and was traditionally believed to improve failing memory. Externally, the essential oil is good for arthritis, rheumatism, and some sorts of headache.

Rumex crispus
YELLOW DOCK

A common hedgerow weed, yellow dock takes its name from its root rather than its nondescript flowers. It was traditionally included in spring tonics, which were gentle laxative and nutritive mixes, taken to combat the effects of a poor winter diet. Today it is a useful digestive remedy that is also used as a cleansing herb for a range of toxic conditions.

Root

Fresh plant

PARTS USED: Root.

KEY USES: The herb is a cleanser for conditions like eczema, as well as for arthritis and rheumatism. It is also a mild laxative and digestive stimulant.

CAUTION:
• Excessive use may lead to diarrhea.

Fresh flowers

Salvia officinalis
SAGE

Like other herbs associated with "women's problems," a thriving sage bush in the garden was believed to show that "the mistress was master" and ruled the house. Drinking sage infusions regularly was recommended for a long life and the herb was once regarded as a panacea and general tonic.

Fresh aerial parts

Essential oil

Dried aerial parts

PARTS USED: Leaves, essential oil.

KEY USES: Sage's actions tend to focus on the mouth, throat, and female reproductive system, and it is used to treat ailments from mouth ulcers to menopausal sweats. Like many culinary herbs it is also a good digestive remedy, stimulating bile flow and regulating its action. Externally, sage is useful as a hair rinse and ointment for insect bites.

CAUTIONS:
• Avoid taking high doses in pregnancy.
• Sage should not be taken by epileptics.

Sambucus nigra
ELDER

Once known as "nature's medicine chest" because of the usefulness of its various parts, only the elder's flowers are widely used today, although herbalists sometimes still make traditional "green ointment" from the young stems and leaves. The tree is common in the countryside, and its rich purple berries are ideal for making winter wine or jam.

PARTS USED: Flowers.

KEY USES: Elderflowers are excellent for all sorts of phlegm-associated conditions, including colds, flu, and hay fever. They reduce fevers and inflammations and can be used both internally and externally. The berries are a palatable source of vitamin C.

Schisandra chinensis
SCHIZANDRA/WU WEI ZI

One of the most popular tonic herbs in China, schizandra berries are well known as an aphrodisiac and were once also taken regularly by wealthy Chinese women to beautify the skin. The Chinese name, *Wu Wei Zi*, means "five taste fruit" although the predominant flavor is actually quite sour.

Dried fruit

Fresh plant

PARTS USED: Fruit.

KEY USES: Schizandra is a good all-around relaxing tonic, useful for insomnia and anxiety. It can also live up to its reputation as a sexual invigorator. The herb can be helpful in allergic or irritant skin conditions, and can also be added to cough remedies.

Scutellaria lateriflora
SKULLCAP

Virginian skullcap arrived in Europe in the 17th century from the US and was known as "mad dog herb" from its reputation as a remedy for rabies. Today, the herb is used for nervous disorders with the native European species, *S. galericulata*, reputedly having similar properties. The name derives from the scoop-shaped seed pods that resemble skullcaps.

PARTS USED: Aerial parts.

KEY USES: It is an excellent sedative and antispasmodic, ideal for all sorts of nervous tension, anxiety, overexcitability, insomnia and stress-related problems.

Fresh aerial parts

Dried aerial parts

Stachys betonica
WOOD BETONY

One of the most popular medieval herbs, wood betony was at one time recommended for almost everything from insanity to prostate problems. It was often worn as an amulet to ward off disease and was recommended in the *Grete Herbal* of 1516 for "those that are fearful." Uncommon in herb gardens today, it is a very pretty plant, with bright pink flowers in midsummer.

PARTS USED: Aerial parts.

KEY USES: Today, wood betony is mostly used as a sedative and as a digestive remedy. It has a tonic effect on the circulation, especially in the brain, making it useful for headaches and as a tonic for the elderly.

CAUTION:
• Avoid high doses in pregnancy.

Fresh aerial parts

Dried aerial parts

Tanacetum parthenium
FEVERFEW

Early herbalists, like John Parkinson in the 17th century, believed feverfew was far too bitter to eat raw and recommended frying the leaves first. Today, it is an extremely popular remedy for migraine. It is commonly grown as a garden plant and can be confused with chamomile.

Fresh flowers

Fresh plant

PARTS USED: Leaves.

KEY USES: Taken regularly, feverfew can reduce the risk and severity of migraine attacks. It is also strongly anti-inflammatory and can be helpful in rheumatoid arthritis. The tea can be taken for menstrual pain.

CAUTIONS:
• Fresh feverfew can occasionally trigger mouth ulcers. Stop taking the herb if this happens. • Feverfew should not be taken by those taking warfarin or similar anticlotting remedies.

Taraxacum officinale
DANDELION

Dandelion's country name of "piddley bed" testifies to its traditional use as a potent diuretic. It is a relatively recent arrival to the herbal repertoire, known to be used medicinally in Europe only since the 15th century. Although the herb is usually classed as a weed, the young leaves are good to eat in salads.

Fresh flower

Fresh root

Fresh leaf

PARTS USED: Leaves, root.

KEY USES: The leaves, which are rich in potassium, are a more potent diuretic than the root. The latter makes an excellent liver tonic, useful for a variety of digestive complaints. The herb is also a good cleanser for skin and arthritic problems.

Thymus vulgaris
THYME

Thyme is an excellent antiseptic herb for the respiratory system and for centuries has been used for treating bronchitis and troublesome coughs. Some scholars argue that the name comes from a Greek word meaning "courage," because the herb is such a stimulating tonic.

PARTS USED: Aerial parts, essential oil.

KEY USES: As well as being an important respiratory remedy, thyme is a good digestive herb, warming and astringent for nausea and diarrhea. The oil is extremely antiseptic and healing and may be applied well diluted directly to wounds.

CAUTION:
•Avoid high doses in pregnancy.

Dried aerial parts

Fresh aerial parts

Essential oil

Urtica dioica
STINGING NETTLE

Gardeners may condemn stinging nettles as "robbing the soil" of nutrients but their greedy feeding helps concentrate a wealth of minerals and vitamins in the plant, making it an ideal remedy for many deficiency problems. Some nettle varieties were spread through Europe by the Romans who used them as a warming, if painful, body rub in cold climates and until recently "urtication," or beating with nettles, was a standard folk remedy for arthritis and rheumatism.

PARTS USED: Aerial parts.

KEY USES: A circulatory stimulant and diuretic, stinging nettles are often used for treating irritant skin conditions. They also clear uric acid from the system, thereby relieving gout and arthritis. The nutrient-rich leaves of stinging nettles make a useful tonic for general use or in anemia.

Dried aerial parts

Tilia europaea
LINDEN

The linden, or lime, tree is a familiar sight, growing on streets in many European cities, with characteristic winged seeds that appear in autumn. The tea is popular in Europe, where it is often known by its French name *tilleul,* and is drunk as a soothing after-dinner infusion.

PARTS USED: Flowers.

KEY USES: Linden is a useful sedative for nervous tension and anxiety. It helps reduce the buildup of fatty deposits in blood vessels (atherosclerosis) and relaxes the blood vessels, making it a particularly good remedy for high blood pressure associated with stress. The herb is also helpful in fevers.

Fresh plant

Fresh aerial parts

Verbena officinalis
VERVAIN

Once sacred to the Druids, vervain was used in fortune-telling and witchcraft well into the 17th century. Traditionally, it was gathered during the "dog days" in July for maximum potency. The original species is a drab, weedy plant, but related ornamental varieties are widely available.

PARTS USED: Aerial parts.

KEY USES: Vervain is a good liver stimulant and a relaxing nerve tonic and is used for a range of digestive problems, as well as depression and tension. It can also be used to ease labor pains, to alleviate various skin conditions, and is regarded as spiritually uplifting.

CAUTION:
• Avoid high doses in pregnancy.

Fresh aerial parts

Dried aerial parts

Viola tricolor
HEARTSEASE

This herb was once a favorite addition to love potions, hence its common name, while the Ancient Greeks used it to reduce anger and soothe headaches. The plant was considered to symbolize pleasant thoughts. It also has a long history as a respiratory remedy.

PARTS USED: Aerial parts

KEY USES: Heartsease is a useful expectorant for chest coughs and can be helpful for a wide range of infected or inflamed skin conditions. It is a mild, cleansing diuretic and contains rutin, which is a good restorative for capillary membranes.

Powder

Fresh aerial parts

Zea mays
CORNSILK

Indian corn, or maize, was once the staple food of many Native American tribes, vital in the diet and also used as a medicine. Ground corn was used by the Aztecs for dysentery and urinary infections, and the early European settlers were quick to recognize its importance.

PARTS USED: Stamens.

KEY USES: The fine, silky stamens are mainly used as a soothing diuretic, for irritant bladder conditions like cystitis, and for prostate problems. It can sometimes be helpful for bedwetting children.

Dried stamens

Zingiber officinalis
GINGER

An important Chinese herb, ginger has been used in the West for more than 2,000 years, both medicinally and in cooking. Traditionally, it was added to many complex remedies to reduce toxicity or side-effects. It is a tropical plant but in cooler climates can be grown in conservatories or greenhouses.

PARTS USED: Root, essential oil

KEY USES: A very warming herb, ideal for colds and chills or as a circulatory stimulant. It helps reduce nausea, so can be taken for travel or morning sickness. It is also a calming digestive remedy, reducing gas and indigestion.

Essential oil

Fresh root

GROWING HERBS & MAKING REMEDIES

FORMER GENERATIONS took growing herbs and making remedies for granted. They knew just what to mix and how to concoct herbal preparations to treat everyday ailments. Today, many Westerners have lost these skills, and though brewing herbal teas and making tonic wines may sound like culinary activities, preparing ointments or tinctures can seem daunting to the uninitiated. However, all herbal remedies are simple to make. In this section, guidelines are given for growing, harvesting, and storing herbs, followed by detailed, step-by-step instructions on how to make many different types of herbal remedies, with a guide to herbs commonly found in over-the-counter preparations.

GROWING HERBS

THERE IS NOTHING MORE pleasant than being able to snip a few herbs from your own garden or window box for a therapeutic tea or a healing ointment. Homegrown and freshly dried herbs have the advantage of being far more potent than commercially grown herbs, which may have been stored for many months before sale, and, for the less common medicinal herbs, home cultivation is often the most practical way to ensure a constant supply of plants. Growing herbs is not difficult and there are many varieties that look very attractive, as well as providing a constant array of delightful and healing aromas to enjoy within the garden.

The medicinal herb garden

Most gardens boast an impressive variety of medicinal plants. There can be hardly any, for example, that do not have shepherd's purse, cleavers, dandelion, stinging nettle, or chickweed lurking in some weedy corner – all of which have valuable therapeutic properties. In addition, many of the commonly grown culinary herbs, such as basil, sage, thyme, and parsley, may be used medicinally.

Some important therapeutic plants, however, such as chamomile, hyssop, and wood betony are unlikely to be found in the garden by chance, and have to be cultivated. It is also worthwhile to consider growing wild flowers in the herb garden, such as agrimony, meadowsweet,

The distinctive yellow spikes of mullein growing in a medicinal herb garden.

melilot, and St.-John's-wort, partly for convenience and also because the roadsides where they grow wild may be polluted.

When planning a herb garden, it is important to take account of the size that chosen plants will grow to, and whether they prefer light or shade. A common misconception is that herbs are drab plants, but it is possible to buy variegated and unusual varieties to add color and interest. If you are planting medicinal herbs for the first time, try the ten herbs listed at the right. Other easily grown plants that are particularly useful include: garlic, heartsease, lady's mantle, marjoram, mullein, peppermint, rosemary, self-heal, vervain, and yarrow.

Helpful houseplants

Potted plants have been grown in homes for centuries, but modern research has revealed a new use for them: it has been shown that many plants absorb polluting chemicals from the atmosphere, converting them to harmless substances. Growing plants in downtown offices or inner-city homes can therefore help improve the environment for the people who live or work there.

Spider plants, common ivy, azaleas, weeping figs, peace lilies, aloe vera, and many other common house plants are reputed to absorb a wide variety of pollutants such as formaldehyde, benzene, and trichloroethylene from the atmosphere. Basil, sage, thyme, oregano, and rosemary can freshen the air around you. These and other plants can be helpful in keeping your living or working spaces fresh and clean.

Planting a herb garden

The ten useful herbs below will make a good basis for a medicinal herb garden. For general guidelines on growing and harvesting herbs, see pp. 52–7.

Chamomile The flowers can be used to make a delicious and soothing infusion to encourage sleep and ease indigestion.

Fennel A dramatic centerpiece for the garden. Collect the seeds for digestive complaints.

Hyssop An attractive, low-growing shrub. Harvest the aerial parts during summer to use in remedies for chest and digestive ailments.

Lemon balm Use the leaves for a restoring and antidepressant tea. Note: This plant self-seeds prolifically and can get out of hand.

Pot marigold An astringent, healing herb; taken internally for digestive problems or mouth ulcers. It can also be applied externally in creams to treat skin disorders.

Purple sage The leaves are used in mouthwashes. Protect with straw or sacking during harsh winters.

Rosemary Use to make hot infused oils for arthritis. Protect young plants with sacking in winter.

St.-John's-wort Use the fresh flowers to make an infused oil that is invaluable for treating burns and inflammations. Harvest during midsummer and use the leaves to make a relaxing tea.

Skullcap A sedative for stress and tension. Harvest during flowering when the distinctive skullcap-shaped pods are forming.

Thyme This is one of the best antiseptics in the herbal repertoire. It is useful for lung infections, as a digestive tonic and as a mouthwash.

Medicinal window box

Apartment-dwellers and those with small gardens may like to plant medicinal herbs in a window box. Herbs will grow happily for one or two seasons in containers, but fresh planting each spring is recommended to ensure healthy plants. Herbs thrive in poor soil and a soil-based potting mix is suitable. If using a peat-based mix add one part grit to five parts potting mix to improve soil texture and drainage.

MEDICINAL WINDOW BOX Choose slow-growing varieties of herbs and look out for some of the attractive variegated varieties available. Plant the taller herbs at the back and put trailing plants near the edge.

PEPPERMINT *leaves may be used in teas for indigestion, nausea, and headaches.*

LEMON BALM *has a wonderful aroma and tastes good in teas. Choose the variegated variety that retains the plant's medicinal properties but will not grow as vigorously.*

WOOD BETONY *adds color to the window box and the leaves can be collected to make a relaxing tea to counteract stress and tension.*

PURPLE SAGE *is a must; it is used in gargles for sore throats, hair rinses, and teas. A slow-growing herb, it is suitable for window boxes.*

THYME *eases coughs and chest complaints and is useful in mouthwashes.*

ROMAN CHAMOMILE *is a low-growing perennial that will provide a steady stream of flowers throughout summer for tea-making.*

SELF-HEAL *is an attractive plant, useful in eyewashes for inflamed or tired eyes.*

GROUND IVY *is a very useful decongestant for colds. Use the leaves in infusions or tinctures.*

Buying plants

Although it is always satisfying to grow herbs from seeds or cuttings, some herbs are slow-growing or difficult to propagate, in which case it is well worth buying plants to help establish the herb garden quickly. A visit to a good specialist nursery also reveals a wide range of decorative varieties of herbs: it is worth looking for variegated lemon balm and mugwort, red ribwort plantain, and the various pink, white, and blue-flowered varieties of hyssop, lavender, and rosemary, all of which can help add a dash of color to the herb garden.

■ Look for strong, healthy specimens with plenty of new growth and space in the pot for expansion.

Straggly, yellowing herbs will give disappointing results when planted in the garden.

■ Examine plants for pests: spider mite, aphids, and whitefly tend to congregate on the underside of leaves or on new growth.
■ Check on roots and potting practices by upturning the pot and tapping it gently so that the plant slides out. Healthy root growth should be evident and the potting mix should hold its shape.
■ Check that plants are correctly labeled. Try to have some idea of what the plant should look like before

buying, and if you are unsure ask nursery staff to check.
■ Most specialist herb nurseries expect a peak in sales in mid- to late spring and will gear production to these times. It is advisable to buy herbs at this time of year, since later in the season plants are likely to become pot-bound. Good nurseries will regularly pot up their products to larger containers as the season progresses, but the price of the herbs usually rises accordingly.

Growing from seed

It is not worth buying annual herbs in pots – like other annuals, they are far better grown from seed. With patience, many perennial herbs may be grown from seed too, although taking cuttings or dividing established plants is sometimes more efficient.

■ Seeds for common medicinal herbs are generally available from garden centers – bear in mind that some, such as melilot and wood betony, will probably be sold in the

wild flower section. Specialist herb nurseries can help with hard-to-find seeds.
■ Most annual herbs should be sown in spring, directly where they are intended to grow. Perennials fare better

if sown in late summer, potted, and kept in a greenhouse during the winter, before being planted out in the spring.
■ Annual medicinal and salad herbs to sow regularly include: anise, basil, borage, California poppy, coriander, corn salad, dill, German chamomile, nasturtium, pot marigold, and salad arugula.

■ Although a biennial, parsley is best sown annually – ideally in the place where it is intended to grow. Other biennials to grow from seed include angelica, melilot, and mullein.
■ Perennial herbs to grow from seed include: elecampane, fennel, fever-few, hyssop, lady's mantle, sage, St.-John's-wort, self-heal, skullcap, and thyme.

SOWING SEEDS

Pot marigold seedling

Glass

Seeds

Widger

1 Fill a seedtray with well-watered potting mix. Sprinkle on the seeds. Cover large seeds with a fine layer of mix (do not cover small seeds). Cover the tray with glass. Alternatively, place the tray in a plastic bag and store in a warm place (up to 68°F/20°C).

2 Fill a pot with potting mix. Gently pick up a seedling with a widger, insert it in a small hole in the mix, and pack the soil around it.

Pruning & controlling

Some herbs grow rapidly and need vigorous pruning and controlling. In medicinal herb cultivation, regular cropping of plant material to dry for future use usually limits the need to do too much pruning. In general, cut herbaceous herbs back to 4–6 in (10–15 cm) high when collecting aerial parts. Where only specific parts of a plant are used (e.g. lavender flowers), normal gardening rules for pruning apply.

■ Prune rosemary, sage, and lavender after flowering, cutting back to 4–8 in (10–20 cm) of new growth.
■ Self-seeders such as fever-few, lady's mantle, lemon balm, mullein and skullcap will colonize the entire garden if not controlled.

■ Some herbs such as mint and soapwort grow so rapidly that they choke other plants. Confine to small areas of the garden.
■ Avoid pruning rue on damp sunny days because this can cause skin rashes. Clip after flowering.

PRUNING HERBS

Lavender

1 Using pruners, cut the dead flower stalks to 4–8 in (10–20 cm) of new growth in late summer or early autumn.

2 Early the following spring, cut back shoots by 1 in (2.5 cm). Ensure that some green growth remains.

Root division

Many herbs are best propagated by root division. Use a small fork to lever clumps of chives apart in autumn and divide lovage roots with a sharp spade in the early spring when growth has just started. Replant after division and water thoroughly. Other herbs propagated in this way include lemon balm and thyme. To propagate elecampane, Roman chamomile, and peppermint, take the runners they develop and replant.

Taking cuttings

Woody perennial herbs are best propagated by cuttings rather than seed. Cuttings can be selected from the side shoots of bushy herbs like sage or rosemary, when semiripe in late summer or early autumn, or from the new softwood growth in spring and early summer when growth must develop quickly if the cutting is to survive. Using semiripe cuttings is usually more successful for medicinal herbs such as elder, hyssop, lavender, lemon verbena, rosemary, purple sage, and thyme.

TAKING CUTTINGS

1 Select a suitable shoot. Break or cut it off, keeping a heel of the main stem attached if possible.

Rosemary cutting

Heel

2 Dip the base of the cutting in hormone rooting powder.

Hormone rooting powder

Dibber

3 Fill a 4 in (10 cm) pot with potting mix. Make a hole with a dibber and insert a seedling. Insert further seedlings until the pot is filled. Water well. After a few weeks roots should appear at the base of the pot. Repot the individual cuttings into 3–4 in (75–100 cm) pots.

HARVESTING & DRYING HERBS

SEASONAL GROWING PATTERNS mean that it is not possible to use fresh herbs throughout the year. Crops have to be harvested, dried, and stored for use when fresh plants are unavailable. Herbs should always be dried as quickly as possible to prevent valuable aromatic chemicals from evaporating and to limit oxidization of important constituents.

The time when herbs are harvested can affect the composition of active chemicals. In many cultures complex rites accompany the gathering of medicinal herbs, which are, in part, associated with magical traditions, but which also frequently ensure that herbs are harvested when they are most potent.

Herbs should be collected on a dry day, after the dew has dried, at the peak of maturity when the concentration of active ingredients is at its highest. Dry them quickly away from bright sunlight, allowing plenty of air to circulate. An airing cupboard with the door open is ideal; otherwise a warm room where they will be undisturbed is suitable. A dry garden shed with a low-powered fan running can be used, but it is not advisable to use a garage, since herbs may become contaminated by gasoline fumes. Keep the area in which the herbs are dried at 70-90° F/ 20-32° C. Most herbs can be dried completely within 5–6 days, although seeds take longer. It is not recommended to dry herbs in a microwave oven. Some researchers have found that this sort of radiation can transform the chemicals in herbs into other substances.

When to harvest

Most herbs are harvested in the summer, either before or during flowering. Seeds and bark are collected in early autumn, and roots in early autumn or spring. The leaves of evergreens such as rosemary, sage, and thyme can be collected at any time (but do not gather large amounts when there is a risk of frost).

—————— EARLY SPRING ——————
Roots: dandelion.

—————— LATE SPRING ——————
Aerial parts during flowering: lungwort, sweet violet.
Flowers: coltsfoot, cowslip, elder.

—————— EARLY TO MIDSUMMER ——————
Aerial parts/leaves before flowering: agrimony, angelica, catnip, cleavers, dandelion, dill, fennel, feverfew, garlic, hyssop, lady's mantle, lemon balm, motherwort, parsley, peppermint, plantain, sage, stinging nettles, white horehound, yellow dock.
Bark while flowering: cramp bark.
Flowers/flowering tops: borage, chamomile, honeysuckle, linden, pot marigold, St.-John's-wort.

—————— MID- TO LATE SUMMER ——————
Aerial parts while flowering: California poppy, heartsease, marjoram, marshmallow, meadowsweet, melilot, mugwort, shepherd's purse, skullcap, thyme, vervain, wild lettuce, wood betony, wormwood, yarrow.
Flowers: hops, lavender, mullein.
Leaves after flowering: borage, coltsfoot, cowslip, fenugreek, lungwort, sweet violet.

—————— AUTUMN ——————
Roots/bulbs when leaves have wilted: angelica (first year), black cohosh, burdock (first year), comfrey, cowslip, elecampane (2–3 year-old roots), garlic, goldenseal, lovage, marshmallow, purple coneflower, soapwort, tormentil, valerian.
Seeds/fruit when ripe: bitter orange, celery, dill, elder, fennel, fenugreek, hawthorn, lovage.

Flowers

Flowerheads are generally gathered when the plant is in full bloom (see p. 54), and are usually dried whole. Gather them in the morning when they are fully open, after the morning dew has dried. Carefully cut each flowerhead off the stalk, remove any insects or dirt, and place on a tray lined with absorbent paper. Small flowers, such as lavender, are dried in the same way as seeds – by hanging them upside down and collecting the flowers in a paper bag.

DRYING FLOWERS

1 Carefully place each flowerhead on a paper-lined tray – it does not matter if they are touching. Leave to dry in a warm place – an airing cupboard is ideal – and turn regularly.

Pot marigold flowers

2 When the flowers are completely dry, store in a dark, airtight container. If using pot marigolds, remove the dried petals from the central part of the flower before storing.

Lavender flowers – dry on the stem in a paper bag

Aerial parts & leaves

Gather leaves of deciduous herbs just before flowering and evergreen herbs, such as rosemary, throughout the year (see p. 54). Large leaves, such as burdock, can be harvested and dried individually; smaller leaves, such as lemon balm, are best dried on the stem. If using all the aerial parts, harvest when the plant is flowering, giving a mixture of leaves, stems, flowers, and seedheads.

DRYING AERIAL PARTS & LEAVES

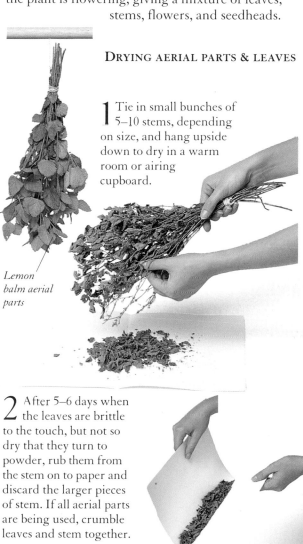

1 Tie in small bunches of 5–10 stems, depending on size, and hang upside down to dry in a warm room or airing cupboard.

Lemon balm aerial parts

2 After 5–6 days when the leaves are brittle to the touch, but not so dry that they turn to powder, rub them from the stem on to paper and discard the larger pieces of stem. If all aerial parts are being used, crumble leaves and stem together.

3 Pour or spoon the dried herbs from the paper into a dark, airtight storage container.

Seeds

Seeds are usually harvested in the early autumn (see p. 54). When the seeds are nearly ripe, cut the seed heads with about a 6–8 in (15–20 cm) stalk, tie them in small bundles with string, and hang them upside down over a paper-lined tray. The seeds fall off when they are dry.

DRYING SEEDS

Fennel seeds

Berries

Berries are harvested when they are just ripe, in the early autumn, before they have become too soft to dry effectively. Spread on paper-lined trays, discarding any that show signs of mold. Preheat the oven and then turn it off, placing the trays in the cooling oven with the door ajar for 3–4 hours. Transfer the trays to an airing cupboard or warm room, turning the berries at regular intervals to ensure even drying.

DRYING BERRIES

Hawthorn berries

Roots

Except for dandelion roots, which are harvested in spring, roots are gathered in the autumn, when the aerial parts have died down and before the ground becomes hard, making digging difficult. After they have dried completely, some roots reabsorb moisture from the atmosphere, so it is important to check them regularly and discard any that become soft.

DRYING ROOTS

1 Wash the roots thoroughly to remove soil and dirt. Chop large roots into small pieces to speed up the drying process.

Marshmallow root

2 Spread out the root pieces on a paper-lined tray. Preheat the oven and then turn it off. Put the roots into the cooling oven, leaving the door ajar, for 2–3 hours (4–6 hours for larger roots). Transfer to a warm room or airing cupboard until dry.

Bulbs

Bulbs should be dug up after after flowering when the aerial parts have died down. Collect garlic cloves quickly since they tend to sink downward once the leaves have wilted and can be difficult to find.

Bark

To avoid damaging the plant or tree, bark should be harvested in the autumn when the sap is falling. Never remove all the bark or even a strip of bark completely surrounding a tree. Dust or wipe bark to remove moss or insects, trying not to get it too wet, and then break it up into pieces about 1–2 in (2–5 cm) square. Spread the bark pieces on paper-lined trays and leave to dry in an airing cupboard or warm room.

Sap & gel

Sap may be collected from a variety of plants and trees. To collect sap from a tree, make a deep incision with a knife or drill a hole into the bark and then, depending on how much liquid is expected, tie a cup or bucket to the tree to collect the sap. Sap should be collected only in the autumn to minimize damage to the tree. Sap may also be taken from latex plants such as wild lettuce and greater celandine; simply squeeze the plant over a bowl. (It is a good idea to wear protective gloves since some saps are corrosive.) The gel from the *Aloe vera* plant is very useful in first aid (see p. 136) and can also be used to make creams.

COLLECTING GEL

1 Carefully slice along the center of a leaf and peel back the edges.

2 Using the blunt edge of a knife, scrape the gel from the leaf.

Aloe vera gel

Freezing herbs

It is possible to freeze small quantities of medicinal herbs, but the method is more suitable for culinary herbs. Freeze whole sprigs of fennel or parsley and basil leaves in plastic bags.

Buying dried herbs

It is not always possible to grow all the herbs needed for medicinal use – garden space may be limited and some herbs do not thrive in all climates – so buying dried herbs is often necessary.

- Always buy the minimum quantity you need to avoid unnecessary storage.
- Steer clear of shops that sell herbs from clear glass jars in direct sunlight, or shops where the herbs look as if they have been on the shelves for a long time. Herbs tend to lose their color with age and poor storage, and drab, dusty-looking herbs are a sign that they are well past their prime.
- Poorly harvested and stored herbs can easily become contaminated: check for mouse droppings, signs of mold, insect infestation, or excessive amounts of other plant material – dried grass mixed with eyebright, for example.
- Try to check that herbs are correctly labeled – mistakes do happen. Some herbs have obvious visual clues (look for the characteristic seedpods in skullcap and shepherd's purse, for example), and others have distinctive smells. Buy from a reputable shop or specialist mail order supplier, and get some idea of what the herb should look like before buying.

Storing herbs

Herbs should be stored in airtight, dry containers in cool conditions away from direct sunlight. Most will keep for 12 months with little deterioration. Dark glass or pottery containers are preferable; if using clear glass containers, keep them in a dark cupboard away from the light. Inspect herbs regularly for any signs of mold or insect infestation, including eggs and chrysalises – a common problem especially with organically grown or imported herbs. Label dried herbs with details of variety, source, and date. Note: For information on how to store herbal preparations (infusions, tinctures, creams, ointments, etc.), see pp. 62–79.

HERBAL TEAS

HERBAL INFUSIONS, OFTEN known as herbal "teas," are not only taken to treat specific ailments. They also make delicious and healthy alternatives to tea or coffee for regular drinking during the day or after meals. Herb teas have a wide range of flavors, and it is worth experimenting to discover a mix you enjoy. Fresh herbs may be dried at home for teas, and ready-made teabags are available from health food and grocery stores. Many of the commercial blends, however, depend on fruit peel and berries for flavor and can be very rich in sugar; they are best avoided in some conditions, such as candidiasis. For step-by-step instructions on making herbal teas, see p. 64.

Karkade

In the Middle East, travelers are often welcomed with a glass of "karkade," a cleansing, cooling tea made from hibiscus flowers.

~ INGREDIENTS ~

50 g dried hibiscus petals
25 g sugar or honey
2 litres water

~ HOW TO MAKE THE TEA ~

Soak the petals in 1 liter of cold water for 1–2 hours and then heat to boiling point. Strain and reserve the liquid. Return the petals to the pan adding 1 liter of fresh water and again bring to a boil. Strain and combine the 2 petal extracts adding the sugar or honey. Karkade is traditionally served chilled but it may also be drunk hot.

Karkade

Uplifting tea

A restoring brew to improve well-being and happiness, with herbs traditionally believed to lift the spirits.

~ INGREDIENTS ~

25 g dried chamomile flowers
50 g dried vervain
50 g dried peppermint leaves
50 g dried & crushed linden flowers
25 g dried lavender flowers
25 g dried lemon balm leaves
water

Uplifting tea

~ HOW TO MAKE THE TEA ~

Mix the herbs and store in a dark jar. Place 1–2 teaspoons in a tisane cup or small teapot, add a cup of freshly boiled water and steep for 5–10 minutes. Strain.

Nightcap tea

A hot infusion of relaxing herbs can be just the thing to guarantee a good night's sleep. This mixture is adapted from a recipe of the great French herbalist, Maurice Mességué.

~ INGREDIENTS ~

25 g dried California poppies
50 g dried wild lettuce leaves
25 g dried hawthorn flowers
25 g dried melilot
water

Nightcap tea

~ HOW TO MAKE THE TEA ~

Mix and store the herbs. Place 1–2 teaspoons in a tisane cup or small teapot, add a cup of freshly boiled water and steep for 5–10 minutes. Strain. Drink hot before going to bed.

Morning tea

This combination contains stimulating and digestive herbs to provide a refreshing and reviving start to the day.

~ INGREDIENTS ~

25 g dried peppermint leaves
50 g dried hibiscus flowers
50 g dried & crushed strawberry leaves
25 g dried & crushed raspberry leaves
25 g dried marigold petals
25 g dried chamomile flowers
25 g dried cornflowers
water

~ HOW TO MAKE THE TEA ~

Mix and store the herbs in a dark glass or ceramic jar. Place 1–2 teaspoons in a tisane cup or small teapot, add a cup of freshly boiled water and steep for 5–10 minutes. Strain. Drink first thing in the morning.

Morning tea

Relaxing mixture

Try this calming mixture of sedating and calming herbs to help unwind after a hard day's work.

~ INGREDIENTS ~

50 g dried lemon balm leaves
50 g dried chamomile flowers
50 g dried & crushed linden flowers
water

~ HOW TO MAKE THE MIXTURE ~

Mix the herbs and store in a dark jar. Place 1–2 teaspoons in a tisane cup or small teapot. Add a cup of freshly boiled water and steep for 5–10 minutes. Strain.

Relaxing mixture

Herbal teabags

Many herbs are available ready-packed in teabags. Although the flavor is generally not as good as using freshly dried or homegrown herbs, teabags are a convenient option for traveling or for use at work. The following are often available:

CHAMOMILE – very relaxing, carminative, and soothing. Fresh flowers have a potent and pungent flavor, but the dried herb can be disappointing. If the taste is offensive, combine with a little standard Indian tea.

ELDERFLOWER – can be an acquired taste; the herb is effective as a decongestant or for hay fever sufferers.

FENNEL – ideal as an after-dinner tea for those prone to indigestion.

LEMON BALM – a good uplifting herb to give a refreshing start to the day. It is sometimes combined with fennel in commercial products to soothe the digestion.

LINDEN – makes a relaxing after-dinner infusion, often combined with peppermint to improve the flavor.

PASSIONFLOWER – usually combined with other herbs, such as linden or chamomile, to make an effective night-time brew.

PEPPERMINT – a popular herbal tea that can help indigestion and head colds. Do not use to excess (follow the instructions on the package) since peppermint can be an irritant.

ROSEHIP & HIBISCUS – a popular commercial combination that is very cooling and refreshing in hot weather.

VERVAIN – a good liver stimulant and soothing for the nerves; popular after dinner – especially in France. Commercial teabags often combine this herb with peppermint.

WOOD BETONY – a very drinkable herb tea that is soothing and relaxing.

Ready-made teabags

SALAD HERBS

FOR THE MEDIEVAL HOUSEWIFE a "green salad," made with highly flavored salad herbs and raw sliced vegetables, was a popular dish, that also acted as as a tonic for digestions made sluggish by a poor winter diet. Today, salad herbs are still widely appreciated for their beneficial properties. They have an extensive range of therapeutic actions: chicory is useful as a bile stimulant and laxative, fennel eases indigestion, watercress is a rich source of minerals and vitamins, and cabbage – once known as the "poor man's medicine chest" – counteracts problems ranging from arthritis to threadworms.

Dandelion leaves

DANDELION
(Taraxacum officinale)
Dandelion leaves are rich in potassium. They are an effective diuretic, often used for fluid retention, as well as being a useful liver and digestive tonic.

Alfalfa shoots

ALFALFA *(Medicago sativa)*
Sprouted alfalfa is rich in calcium, magnesium, phosphorus, potassium, and almost all known vitamins. It is regarded as a cleansing blood purifier in Eastern medicine.

Watercress leaves

WATERCRESS
(Nasturtium officinale)
Rich in minerals and vitamin C, watercress is an ideal tonic for anemia.

Good King Henry leaves

PURSLANE *(Portulaca oleracea)* Purslane is valued for its high level of omega-3 fatty acids, which affect cholesterol levels and reduce the risk of blood clots and heart attacks.

GOOD KING HENRY *(Chenopodium bonus-henricus)*
Good King Henry is a traditional remedy for indigestion. Its leaves can be eaten raw in salads or used like spinach in flans or egg dishes.

Purslane leaves

*Salad
arugula
leaves*

SALAD ARUGULA
(*Eruca vesicaria*)
Both the leaves and
white flowers can be used in
salads, adding a distinctive
peppery flavor. Once regarded
as a cure-all and aphrodisiac, salad
arugula is a useful
source of vitamin C
and is mildly
diuretic.

*Cilantro
leaves*

CILANTRO
(*Coriandrum
sativum*)
Cilantro leaves are a popular Indian
household remedy for digestive upsets
and urinary tract infections.

*Alecost
leaves*

ALECOST, OR COSTMARY (*Tanacetum
balsamita*) Alecost has astringent
properties and is used as a gentle digestive
stimulant. *Caution*: Do not confuse with the
camphor plant, which has similar leaves.

Salad recipes

Salad leaves, vegetables, and herbs can be used in all kinds of
combinations to make salads that will provide a beneficial addition to
meals. Use ordinary lettuce as a base, or for a splash of color, try
radicchio, red lettuce, red cabbage, or red orache. Then add salad herbs
to suit your taste or dietary needs. Salad herbs are often highly flavored
and need to be used in moderation, especially if you are unfamiliar
with the taste. Limit the use of strong digestive stimulants, such as
dandelion, endive, or nasturtium if eating large amounts of salad.

TONIC SALAD

This mix contains herbs that stimulate
the liver and adrenal glands and
also provide plenty of vitamins
and minerals.

~ HOW TO MAKE THE SALAD ~

Use lettuce – cos, Bibb, or
Boston if possible – and a
few alfalfa sprouts. Add the
following leaves roughly
shredded: basil, dandelion,
Good King Henry, and
parsley. Toss in an olive oil
and lemon juice dressing
and decorate with
nasturtium and borage
flowers or chive florettes.

*Basil
leaves* *Borage
flowers* *Dandelion
leaves*

Nasturtium flowers

Good King Henry leaves

Lettuce *Alfafa shoots* *Parsley*

SALAD FOR THE DIGESTION

This salad combines carminative herbs, used
for easing indigestion, with gentle bile
stimulants that give a mild laxative effect
to help regulate the digestive system.

~ HOW TO MAKE THE SALAD ~

Finely slice a fennel bulb
and combine with endive
leaves. Add 1–2 shredded
alecost leaves and a small
handful of lemon balm
leaves. Toss in a dressing
made from olive oil and
lemon juice and decorate
with sesame seeds or
arugula flowers.

Endive leaves

Sesame seeds

*Alecost
leaves*

Fennel

*Lemon
balm
leaves*

MAKING HERBAL REMEDIES

Equipment

■ Use utensils made from cast iron, enamel, glass, pottery, or stainless steel. Use wooden or steel spatulas and palette knives, and plastic or nylon sieves and tea strainers. Do not use aluminum pans, since many foods and herbs absorb this element, which is potentially toxic. Do not store herbal preparations in plastic containers for long periods, as plastic tends to absorb reactive chemicals from many herbs.

■ All equipment should be kept clean and storage bottles should be sterilized before use. If regularly making herbal remedies, use a separate set of utensils in order to avoid contamination with food bacteria. Otherwise, wash everything in very hot water and thoroughly dry all metal pans and spatulas in a hot oven before use. In addition, keep a separate teapot for making herbal infusions.

■ For equipment suppliers, see p. 140.

■ Label all ingredients and remedies clearly.

Weighing & measuring

WEIGHING HERBS Kitchen scales are generally suitable for weighing herbs. Electronic ones are the simplest to use, usually accurate to 0.1 g. If it is difficult to weigh less than 10 g on your scales, double the quantities given for dried herbs in a recipe and divide the mix in half, reserving one half for the next day's use.

MEASURING LIQUIDS Conical or straight-sided measuring cylinders are simple to use (see p. 74). If it is difficult to measure very small amounts of liquid try using a dropper. Twenty drops from a pipette equals approximately 1 ml.

Sterilizing equipment

Many herbal medicines will soon get moldy if nonsterile storage jars and bottles are used. There is rarely a problem with tinctures, since the high alcohol content kills bacteria, but creams and syrups can rapidly deteriorate.

Sterilization preparations sold for home winemaking or for baby's bottles – usually based on sodium metabisulphite or sodium hypochlorite – are ideal. Before use, soak all storage bottles, jars, and lids in a diluted mixture for at least 30 minutes (or as directed on the package). Rinse with freshly boiled water and dry in a hot oven.

Alternatively, wash glass containers thoroughly in freshly boiled water and place in a hot oven (at least 325° F/160° C) for an hour. Handle with care when removing and use when cool. (This is not suitable for plastic containers.)

Cautions

COLLECTING PLANTS If using freshly gathered wild plant material to make herbal remedies, make sure that you have the correct plant by using a botanical field guide, since some plants may be confused: foxglove leaf, for example, is commonly mistaken for comfrey, and alkanet for borage. See also p. 135 for plants to handle with care.

ESSENTIAL OILS Commercially produced essential oils are commonly adulterated with cheap synthetic ingredients. When buying essential oils always opt for a reputable brand name. Do not take essential oils internally unless directed to do so by a professional practitioner.

DOSAGE The standard adult dose given on the following pages must be reduced for children and the elderly. See pp. 128 and 83 for advice. If pregnant, do not take alcoholic tinctures and see the list of herbs to avoid on p. 126.

MEASURING REMEDIES

1 ml = 20 drops 20 ml = 1 tablespoon
5 ml = 1 teaspoon 60–75 ml = 1 sherry glass
10 ml = 1 heaping teaspoon 150 ml =1 teacup or wineglass

SYRUPS

HONEY OR UNREFINED SUGAR can be combined with infusions or decoctions to make syrups. As well as helping to preserve the active plant ingredients, the sweetness is useful for disguising the flavor of some herbs, such as goldenseal. Syrups are frequently used to treat children. Honey has a particularly soothing effect and is often combined with herbs with an expectorant action to make cough syrups.

EQUIPMENT

• *Teapot* • *Saucepan* • *Nylon or plastic sieve* • *Jug* • *Wooden spoon* • *Airtight, sterilized, dark glass bottles with cork stoppers* • *Funnel (optional)*

PARTS USED

Aerial parts, bark, flowers, leaves, roots

STANDARD QUANTITY

Use 500 ml infusion or decoction and 500 g honey or unrefined sugar.

STANDARD DOSAGE

Take 5–10 ml 3 times a day.

STORAGE

Store in sterilized, dark glass bottles with cork stoppers for up to 3 months.

1 Make a 500 ml standard infusion or decoction of your chosen herbs (see pp. 64–7).

This syrup is made from an infusion of hyssop (Hyssopus officinalis) *and warm honey.*

2 Strain the infusion or decoction into a jug and pour into a clean saucepan.

3 For each 500 ml of infusion add 500 g of warm honey or unrefined sugar and stir constantly until dissolved. Simmer gently until the mixture has a syrupy consistency and then remove from the heat and allow to cool.

4 Pour into bottles and seal with a cork stopper. Syrups can ferment and cork stoppers will simply pop out, whereas screw-top bottles can explode.

INFUSIONS

A VERY SIMPLE and popular way of using herbs, infusions may be taken as remedies for specific ailments or just be enjoyed as relaxing and revitalizing teas. An infusion is made in a very similar way to tea, using fresh or dried herbs. The water should have just begun to boil, since vigorously boiling water disperses valuable volatile oils in the steam. Infusions can be made from a single herb or from a combination of herbs, and may be drunk hot or cold. It is best to make them fresh each day.

One cup infusions

It is often more convenient to make a single cup of infusion. These are made either in a small teapot or in a tisane cup (shown here), which are available from specialty outlets.

Lid

Strainer

Cup

Saucer

EQUIPMENT
- *Kettle* • *Glass or ceramic teapot that holds at least 500 ml water*
- *Nylon or plastic tea strainer* • *Teacup*
- *Teaspoon* • *Jug with a lid for storage*

PARTS USED
Leaves, flowers and most aerial parts (dried or fresh)

STANDARD QUANTITY
For most medicinal teas with a therapeutic action, add 25 g dried or 75 g fresh herb to 500 ml water to make 3 doses. If using a combination of herbs, be sure that the total weight of the mixture does not exceed the standard quantity.

STANDARD DOSAGE
Take a teacup or wineglass dose 3 times daily. Repeat doses may be reheated. Add a little honey or unrefined sugar per dose to taste. Reduce the dose for children and the elderly (see pp. 128 & 83).

STORAGE
Store in a covered jug in a cool place or refrigerator for up to 48 hours.

This infusion is made from fresh lemon balm leaves (Melissa officinalis).

1 Warm a teapot with hot water. Add the fresh or dried herb.

2 Pour on hot water that has just boiled. Cover the teapot with the lid and infuse for 10 minutes.

1 Place 2 teaspoonfuls of dried herb in the strainer. Place the strainer in the cup.

Dried herb in the strainer

2 Pour freshly boiled water on to the herbs. Put the lid on and leave the tea to infuse for 10 minutes. Carefully remove the strainer.

Herbal teabags

4 Take a dose, adding honey or a little unsweetened sugar to taste. Strain the rest into a jug, cover, and store in a cool place or refrigerator.

3 Strain the infusion through a tea strainer.

10 cm

Homemade herbal teabags are very useful when traveling or at the office. Place 1–2 teaspoons of herbs on a muslin square and tie it into a small bundle with string. Simply infuse this for 10 minutes in a teacup of freshly boiled water.

DECOCTIONS

THE DECOCTION METHOD is used for tough plant materials, such as barks, berries, or roots, which need a more vigorous extraction than is possible using the infusion method. Decoction involves heating the plant material in cold water, bringing it to a boil and simmering for 20–40 minutes. Combinations of herbs can be mixed together, or herbs may be used singly. The standard quantity, which can be drunk hot or cold, is enough for three doses and should be made fresh each day. As with infusions, decoctions are frequently used as the basis of other remedies, such as syrups.

EQUIPMENT
- *Saucepan (preferably ceramic, enamel, or stainless steel; do not use aluminum)*
- *Nylon or plastic sieve*
- *Jug with a lid for storage*

PARTS USED
Barks, berries, roots (dried or fresh)

STANDARD QUANTITY
Add 30 g dried or 60 g fresh herb to 750 ml of cold water. This reduces to around 500 ml after simmering. If using a combination of herbs, be sure that the total weight of the mixture does not exceed this standard amount.

STANDARD DOSAGE
Take a teacup or wineglass dose 3 times daily. Repeat doses may be reheated. Honey or unrefined sugar may be used to sweeten each dose, or they may be flavored with a little lemon juice. Reduce the dose for children and the elderly (see pp. 128 & 83).

STORAGE
Store in a covered jug in a cool place or refrigerator for up to 48 hours.

Licorice root

Gao Ben

Devil's claw

This decoction is made from dried licorice root (Glycyrrhiza uralensis), dried Gao Ben (Ligusticum sinense), and dried devil's claw (Harpagophytum procumbens).

1 Place the herb in a saucepan and pour over the cold water.

2 Bring to the boil and simmer gently for 20–40 minutes, until the volume has reduced by about one-third.

3 Take the decoction off the heat and strain through a nylon or plastic sieve into a jug.

4 Pour the decoction into a covered jug and store in a cool place or refrigerator.

Mixed decoction/infusion

For remedies that combine bark, berries, or roots with flowers or leaves use the following method.

1 Mix the bark, berries, or roots together in a cast iron, enamel, or stainless steel saucepan and add 750 ml of cold water.

2 Bring to a boil and simmer for 20–40 minutes, or until the volume has reduced by approximately one-third, to make a decoction.

3 Meanwhile, mix the flowers and leaves needed for the remedy and put them in a glass or ceramic teapot.

4 Strain the hot decoction on to the dried herbs in the teapot and leave to infuse for 10–15 minutes.

5 Strain the final mixture into a covered jug and store in a cool place. Take a teacup dose 3 times a day. Sweeten with a little honey or unrefined sugar to taste.

Macerations

There are some herbs, such as valerian root (*Valeriana officinalis*), that are best macerated rather than infused or decoted. Put 25 g of the dried herb in a saucepan. Add 500 ml of cold water and leave in cool place overnight. Strain through a nylon sieve.

Chinese decoctions

In China, herbs are mainly given in decoctions, and they tend to be more highly concentrated than in the West. Up to 150 g of dried herb to a liter of water is used, reduced down to 300–400 ml for 3 doses. The resulting mixture may need to be diluted with water to suit Western palates.

TINCTURES

TINCTURES ARE MADE BY steeping the herb in a mixture of alcohol and water. They should be made individually, and then prepared tinctures may be combined as required. As well as extracting the plant's active ingredients, the alcohol acts as a preservative, and tinctures will keep for up to two years. The liquid is usually composed of 25% alcohol and 75% water, but for some resinous herbs the amount of alcohol is increased to 45%. Commercially prepared tinctures use ethanol, but diluted spirits are suitable for home use: vodka is ideal since it does not contain additives, but rum helps disguise the flavor of less palatable herbs.

TINCTURE RATIOS Tinctures are sometimes recommended for use in ratio form, for example, "take 5 ml of a 1:4 tincture." When making a tincture in ratio form, the proportion used is weight to volume. A 1:4 tincture could be made with 1 kg herb to 4 liters alcohol/water mix, or 100 g herb to 400 ml alcohol/water mix. The units used are immaterial and can be large or small accordingly.

EQUIPMENT

- *Large screw-top jar*
- *Jelly bag or muslin bag* • *winepress*
- *Large jug* • *Sterilized, dark glass bottles with screw caps for airtight storage* • *Funnel (optional)*

PARTS USED

All parts of the plant (dried or fresh)

STANDARD QUANTITY

Use 200 g dried or 600 g fresh herb to 1 liter of alcohol/water mixture (25% alcohol & 75% water – e.g., dilute a 1 liter bottle of 75 proof vodka with 500 ml water). See Cautions for types of alcohol to avoid.

STANDARD DOSAGE

Take 5 ml 3 times a day diluted in a little warm water. A small amount of honey or fruit juice can often improve the flavor. See also Alcohol-reduced tinctures opposite.

STORAGE

Store in dark glass bottles for up to 2 years.

1 Put the herb into a large jar and cover with the alcohol/water mixture. Seal the jar, store in a cool place for 2 weeks, and shake it occasionally.

This tincture is made from cinnamon sticks (Cinnamomum zeylanicum) and a mixture of vodka and water.

2 Fit a muslin bag inside a winepress. Pour the mixture through.

3 Press the mixture through the winepress into a jug. The residue can be added to the garden compost heap.

Alcohol-reduced tinctures

There are times when giving tinctures made from alcohol in the normal way is unsuitable, for example in pregnancy, in gastric or liver inflammation, or when treating children or recovered alcoholics. Adding a small amount (25–50 ml) of almost boiling water to the tincture dose (usually 5 ml) in a cup and allowing it to cool effectively evaporates most of the alcohol, making it safe.

CAUTIONS

• *Industrial alcohol, denatured alcohol (methyl alcohol), and rubbing alcohol (isopropyl alcohol) are all extremely toxic. Do not use in tincture making.*

• *See Alcohol-reduced tinctures (above) for advice on giving tinctures to children, pregnant women, and former alcoholics.*

4 Pour the strained liquid into sterilized, dark glass bottles, using a funnel if necessary.

TONIC WINES

TONIC HERBS STEEPED IN WINE and taken in small, daily doses are used in many parts of the world as regular restoratives. Some commonly used in this way are the Chinese tonic herbs *Dang Gui, Dang Shen, He Shou Wu,* and Korean ginseng. Western herbs, such as elecampane – a good lung tonic for those prone to coughs – can also be used. The easiest way to make a tonic wine is in a vinegar vat, a large ceramic pot with a tap at the bottom, which allows the liquid to be drained off easily. The herbs should always be kept covered with wine, or they may get moldy and the mixture will have to be discarded.

EQUIPMENT

• *Vinegar vat* • *Alternatively, use a jug with a well-fitting lid and pour the daily dose from the top of the mixture, ensuring it is regularly stirred.*

This tonic wine is made with dried Dang Gui *(Chinese angelica – Angelica sinensis) and red wine.*

PARTS USED
All parts of the plant (dried)

STANDARD QUANTITY
Add enough dried herb to fill the vinegar vat at least three-quarters full, and good quality red or white wine to cover the herb completely. Additional wine will be needed to top off the vat.

STANDARD DOSAGE
Take a sherry glass daily.

STORAGE
The tonic wine may be kept for 3–4 months if regularly topped up. Throw the mixture away if the herbs get moldy, and start again.

Vinegar vat

Tap

1 Fill the vat at least three-quarters full with the chosen herb. Pour on enough wine to cover the mixture completely.

2 Leave for 2 weeks, then take a daily dose from the tap at the bottom of the vat. Make sure the herbs always remain covered with wine, and top off the vat regularly.

CAPSULES

HERBS CAN BE TAKEN IN POWDERED form, sprinked on food, stirred in water, or made into capsules, which are preferable for the less palatable herbs as well as convenient for carrying around. It is best to use commercially produced powders, available from specialist suppliers (see p. 140). Two-part gelatin or vegetarian capsules used may also be obtained from specialist outlets.

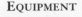

EQUIPMENT
- *Saucer or flat dish*
- *Capsule cases • Dark, airtight containers for storage*

PARTS USED
All parts of the plant
(dried and powdered)

STANDARD QUANTITY
Use 200–250 mg powder to each size 00 gelatin or vegetarian capsule case.

STANDARD DOSAGE
Take 2–3 capsules 2 to 3 times a day.

STORAGE
Store in airtight, dark containers in a cool place for up to 3–4 months.

The capsules are filled with powdered ginger (Zingiber officinalis).

1 Pour the powdered herb into a saucer or flat dish. Separate the 2 halves of a capsule case and slide them together through the powder, scooping it into the capsule.

2 Fit together the 2 halves of the capsule. Store in dark, airtight containers in a cool place.

PESSARIES & SUPPOSITORIES

PESSARIES ARE WAXY pellets containing medication. They are inserted in the vagina and melt at body temperature, delivering the remedy to the site of infection or irritation. Suppositories are similar but intended for anal insertion. They are used when treatments are needed in the lower bowel and medicines taken orally would be broken down during the digestive process. It is best to buy them ready-made. To make pessaries:

1 Use a pessary mold (available from specialist suppliers) or make 24 suitable shapes from cooking foil (1 cm in diameter tapering to 0.5 cm in diameter at one end, and 2 cm in length). Place them on a wire rack. Combine 10 g soft soap, 50 ml glycerine, and 40 ml denatured alcohol to make a lubricant, and pour into the mold or shapes. Leave for a few seconds and pour off the lubricant.

2 Melt 20 g cocoa butter in a double boiler. Remove the pan from the heat and add 30 drops of essential oil. Pour the mixture into the molds and leave to set for about 3 hours. When fully set, open the mold or carefully remove the cooking foil.

3 Store the pessaries in a cool place in a container lined with waxed paper.

Pot marigold & thyme pessaries

COMPRESSES

A COMPRESS IS A cloth soaked in a hot or cold herbal extract. They can be applied to painful joints and muscles, and are useful for soothing skin rashes and irritations. A cold compress is sometimes used for headaches. The cloth may be soaked in an infusion, decoction, or a tincture diluted with hot or cold water. An old tea towel is ideal, or use muslin or cotton wrapped in surgical gauze.

EQUIPMENT
• *Cloth pad* • *Bowl*

STANDARD QUANTITY
Use 500 ml standard infusion or decoction, or 50 ml tincture in 500 ml hot or cold water.

STANDARD APPLICATION
Apply as often as required.

This compress is made with arnica infusion (Arnica montana).

1 Soak a clean piece of soft cloth in a hot infusion or other herbal extract. Squeeze out the excess liquid.

2 Hold the pad against the affected area. When it cools or dries, repeat the process using hot mixture.

POULTICES

A POULTICE OF BREAD or mashed potato soaked in herbal extract was once a favorite household remedy for minor injuries and ailments. Today, poultices are generally made with chopped fresh herbs. They are usually applied hot.

EQUIPMENT
• *Saucepan* • *Gauze/cotton strips*

PARTS USED
Whole plant (dried or fresh) chopped

STANDARD QUANTITY
Use sufficient herb to cover the area.

STANDARD APPLICATION
Apply the poultice every 2–4 hours or more frequently if necessary.

This poultice is made with fresh chopped cabbage leaves (Brassica oleracea).

1 Boil the fresh herb, squeeze out any surplus liquid, and spread it on the affected area. Smooth oil on the skin first, to prevent the herb from sticking.

2 Apply gauze or cotton strips to hold the poultice in place.

HOT INFUSED OILS

ACTIVE PLANT INGREDIENTS can be extracted in oil for external use in massage oils, creams, and ointments. Infused oils will last for up to a year if kept in a cool, dark place, but they are more potent when fresh, so it is best to make small amounts frequently. There are two techniques for making infused oils and the hot method is suitable for leafy herbs such as comfrey, chickweed, stinging nettle, and rosemary.

This hot infused oil is made with dried chickweed (Stellaria media).

EQUIPMENT
• *Glass bowl and saucepan, or double boiler* • *Muslin bag and winepress (or jelly bag)* • *Large jug* • *Airtight, sterilized, dark glass storage bottles* • *Funnel (optional)*

PARTS USED
Aerial parts, leaves (dried)

STANDARD QUANTITY
Use 250 g dried herb to 500 ml sunflower oil.

STORAGE
Store in sterilized, airtight dark glass bottles in a cool place away from direct light for up to a year.

Suitable herbs

Herbs used to make hot infused oils include:
• *Bladderwrack* for arthritic pain.
• *Chickweed* for irritant eczema.
• *Cleavers* for psoriasis.
• *Comfrey* for bruises, sprains, and osteoarthritis.
• *Stinging nettle* for allergic skin rashes and eczema.
• *Rosemary* for aches and pains.

1 Put the oil and the herb in a glass bowl over a pan of simmering water or in a double boiler and heat gently for about 3 hours.

Muslin bag

Winepress

2 Strain the mixture through a muslin bag fitted to a winepress into a jug. Alternatively, strain it through a jelly bag (illustrated on p. 73).

3 Pour the oil into storage bottles, using a funnel if necessary.

COLD INFUSED OILS

THIS METHOD OF MAKING AN infused oil is suitable for flowers such as pot marigold and St.-John's-wort. It is a slow process: the flowers and oil are packed into a jar and left for several weeks, after which the once-infused oil is used again with fresh herb to extract as much active plant ingredient as possible. Cold infused oils are used in massage oils or as the basis for creams or ointments. See below for herbs commonly used in this way.

EQUIPMENT

Large glass screw-top jar • Jelly bag and string (or muslin bag and winepress) • Large jug • Airtight, sterilized, dark glass storage bottles • Funnel (optional)

PARTS USED
Aerial parts, flowers (fresh or dried)

STANDARD QUANTITY
Use double quantities of enough fresh or dried herb to pack a storage jar, and about 1 liter cold-pressed safflower or walnut oil (the quantity will depend on the size of jar used).

STORAGE
Store in sterilized, airtight dark glass bottles in a cool place away from direct light for up to a year.

This cold infused oil is made with fresh St.-John's-wort flowering tops (Hypericum perforatum).

1 Pack a large jar tightly with the herb and cover completely with oil. Put the lid on and leave on a sunny windowsill or in a greenhouse for 2–3 weeks.

Jelly bag

2 Pour the mixture into a jelly bag fitted with string or an elastic band to the rim of a jug. Or use a muslin bag and a winepress (illustrated on p. 72).

3 Squeeze the oil through the bag. Repeat steps 1 and 2 with new herb and the once-infused oil. After a few weeks, strain once more, and pour into storage bottles, using a funnel if necessary.

Suitable herbs

Herbs used to make cold infused oils include:

• *Melilot* (use dried herb) for varicose eczema.

• *Pot marigold* (use fresh or dried petals) for scrapes, dry eczema and fungal infections such as athlete's foot.

• *St.-John's-wort* (use fresh flowering tops) for sunburn, minor scalds and burns, scratches, and inflamed joints.

MASSAGE OILS

MASSAGE OILS ARE MADE from a few drops of essential oil diluted in a carrier oil – sweet almond or wheat germ is best, but sunflower or other vegetable oil may be used. Infused oils are also used as carriers. Once diluted, essential oils soon deteriorate, so it is best to mix small amounts frequently. Massage requires skill and practice, and is not suitable for some conditions (see Cautions below).

PARTS USED
Essential oil

STANDARD QUANTITY
In general, use no more than a 10% concentration of essential oils, i.e., up to 5 ml of essential oil in 45 ml of carrier oil (sweet almond, wheat germ or vegetable oil). Reduce this to a maximum of 5% essential oil for children, the elderly, or those with sensitive skins. Use good-quality essential oil.

STANDARD APPLICATION
Pour about 2–5 ml (½-1 teaspoonful) onto the hands (not directly onto the body) and rub gently.

STORAGE
Store in a sterilized, airtight dark glass bottle in a cool place.

CAUTIONS FOR MASSAGE
- *Pregnant women should seek professional advice and should not use essential oils at all during the first 3 months of pregnancy.*
- *Do not massage anyone suffering from an infection, epilepsy, a contagious disease, acute back pain (especially if the pain shoots down the arms and legs), or from an inflammatory condition such as thrombosis or phlebitis.*
- *Do not massage bruised or inflamed areas.*

EQUIPMENT
- *Small and large graduated cylinders*
- *50 ml sterilized, airtight dark glass bottle • Funnel (optional)*

This massage oil is made with lavender (Lavandula angustifolia) *and thyme* (Thymus vulgaris) *essential oils and wheat germ oil.*

1 Measure out the carrier oil into the large graduated cylinder and the essential oil into the small graduated cylinder, using the funnel if preferred.

Small graduated cylinder (to measure 5 ml)

Large graduated cylinder (to measure 45 ml)

2 Pour the carrier oil and the essential oil into the bottle, using the funnel if necessary.

Measured-out essential oil

3 Shake the bottle well to mix the oils.

OINTMENTS

OINTMENTS CONTAIN oils or fats, but no water. Unlike creams, they do not blend with the skin, but form a separate layer over it. They are suitable where the skin is already weak or soft, or where some protection is needed from additional moisture, as in diaper rash. Ointments were once made from animal fats, but petroleum jelly or paraffin wax is suitable. Infused oils may be used instead of the herb itself (see p. 76).

(see p. 76)

EQUIPMENT

- *Glass bowl and saucepan, or double boiler* • *Wooden spoon* • *Jelly bag and string (or muslin bag and winepress)* • *Jug* • *Rubber gloves* • *Sterilized, airtight dark glass jars with lids*

PARTS USED
All parts of the plant (dried and fresh)

STANDARD QUANTITY
Use 500 g petroleum jelly or soft paraffin wax and 60 g dried or 150 g fresh herb.

STANDARD APPLICATION
Rub a little into the affected part 2–3 times a day.

STORAGE
Store in sterilized, airtight dark jars, for 3–4 months in a cool place.

This ointment is made with dried stinging nettle (Urtica dioica).

1 Melt the jelly or wax in a bowl over a pan of boiling water or in a double boiler. Add the herbs and heat for 2 hours or until the herbs are crisp. Do not allow the pan to boil dry.

2 Pour the mixture into a jelly bag fitted with string or an elastic band to the rim of a jug, or else use a muslin bag and a winepress (see p. 72).

(see p. 72)

3 If using a jelly bag wear rubber gloves, since the mixture is hot. Squeeze the mixture through the jelly bag into the jug.

4 Quickly pour the strained mixture, while still warm and melted, into jars.

Suitable herbs

- *Arnica* for bruises, sprains, and frostbite (only use on unbroken skin).
- *Capsicum* for shingles.
- *Chamomile* for eczema and other allergic skin conditions.
- *Chickweed* for irritant eczema, corns, boils, or splinters.
- *Elderflower* for chapped hands.
- *Heartsease* for rashes.
- *Melilot* for swellings and varicose eczema.
- *Plantain* for dry eczema.
- *Stinging nettle* for haemorrhoids and eczema.

CREAMS

A CREAM IS A MIXTURE of water with fats or oils, which softens and blends with the skin. It can easily be made using emulsifying ointment (available from most pharmacies), which is a mixture of oils and waxes that blends with water or tinctures. Homemade creams will last for several months, but the shelf life is prolonged by storing the mixture in a cool pantry or refrigerator, or adding a few drops of benzoin tincture as a preservative. Creams made from organic oils and fats deteriorate more quickly. The method shown here is suitable for most herbs.

PARTS USED
All parts of the plant
(fresh or dried)

STANDARD QUANTITY
Use 150 g emulsifying ointment,
70 ml glycerol, 80 ml water and
30 g dried or 75 g fresh herb.

STANDARD APPLICATION
Rub a little into the affected part
2–3 times a day.

STORAGE
Store in sterilized, airtight dark jars
for up to 3 months in a cool place.

This cream is made with dried pot marigold (Calendula officinalis).

1 Melt the emulsifying ointment in a double boiler or a bowl over a pan of boiling water. Pour in the glycerol and water and stir well. The mixture will solidify slightly when the liquid is added, so keep the bowl over the boiling water and stir to remelt it.

2 Add the herb and stir well. Simmer for 3 hours, regularly adding more boiling water to the lower saucepan to prevent the pan from burning.

3 Use a winepress or jelly bag fitted to a jug, and strain the hot mixture as quickly as possible into a bowl. Stir the melted, strained cream constantly as it cools, to avoid separation. If it does start to separate, return it to the double boiler and reheat with an additional 10–20 g of emulsifying ointment.

CREAMS & OINTMENTS FROM INFUSED OILS
Creams and ointments can be made using hot and cold infused oils instead of dried herbs. (To make the infused oils, see pp. 72–3.) For a cream, melt 25 g beeswax with 25 g anhydrous lanolin (both available over the counter), add 100 ml infused oil and 50 ml herbal tincture (to make, see p. 68). Strain, stir, and when the cream has set, put into storage jars using a palette knife. To make an ointment, melt 25 g beeswax with 25 g anhydrous lanolin, then add 100 ml infused oil. Pour into sterilized, dark glass jars while still warm, and allow to cool.

4 When the cream has set, use a small palette knife to fill storage jars. Put some cream around the edge of the jar first, and then fill the middle to avoid air bubbles.

LOTIONS & EMULSIONS

A LOTION IS A WATER-BASED mixture, applied to the skin as a cooling or soothing remedy to relieve irritation or inflammation. Alcohol-based mixtures, such as tinctures, may be added to lotions to increase the cooling effect. Emulsions are also water-based mixtures, consisting of oil and water shaken to form a suspension. Both remedies are made in the same way and can be stored in dark glass bottles for up to three months.

EQUIPMENT
- *Graduated cylinder*
- *Sterilized, dark glass storage bottles*
- *Funnel (optional)*

PARTS USED
All parts of the plant
(fresh or dried)

STANDARD QUANTITY
Lotions and emulsions vary in composition depending on use. The lotion featured here is for a skin rash: 40 ml distilled witch hazel, 40 ml rose water, 20 ml chickweed tincture. An emulsion for warts can be made by combining 5 ml tea tree oil and 5 ml thuja tincture.

STANDARD APPLICATION
Lotions and emulsions are usually mild and can be used liberally as required to ease symptoms.

STORAGE
Store in sterilized, dark glass bottles for up to 3 months in a cool place.

This lotion is made with chickweed tincture (Stellaria media).

1 Using a graduated cylinder, measure out the first ingredient.

2 Pour it into the glass bottle using a funnel if necessary. Repeat steps 1 and 2 with the other ingredients.

3 Shake the bottle well.

STEAM INHALATIONS

CONDITIONS SUCH AS sinusitis, bronchitis, or asthma can be relieved with steam inhalations, which clear the respiratory system of excess mucus. Well-diluted infusions or essential oils are used, with active plant ingredients that are anti-allergenic and anti-inflammatory. After treatment, stay in a warm room for 30 minutes to give the airways time to readjust.

This steam inhalation uses chamomile essential oil (Matricaria recutita).

EQUIPMENT
• *Kettle* • *Basin* • *Towel*

PARTS USED
Essential oil or infusion

STANDARD QUANTITY
Add 500 ml of standard infusion (to make, see p. 64) or up to 10 drops of good quality essential oil (see the note on p. 62) to a basin of steaming hot water.

STANDARD DOSAGE
Use once or twice a day, inhaling the steam for 10 minutes each time.

1 Boil water in a kettle and half fill a basin with steaming water. Add 500 ml of standard infusion or 5–10 drops of essential oil (or a mixture of oils).

2 Drape a towel over the head and basin to contain the steam, then inhale steadily for 10 minutes. Breathe normally, rather than too deeply.

BATHS & WASHES

ESSENTIAL OILS CAN BE added to bathwater for a relaxing soak to ease aching limbs, clear stuffy noses, and relieve many other minor ailments. Use 2–5 drops of undiluted essential oil in the bathwater and stir well to disperse the oil. Some of the more useful oils are:
• *Chamomile* for anxiety, insomnia, and period pain.
• *Eucalyptus* for coughs, colds, aches, and pains.
• *Lavender* for headaches, aches, pains, and stress.
• *Peppermint* for fatigue and nasal congestion.
• *Rosemary* for fatigue, aching joints, and period pain.

Footbaths

Footbaths are ideal for relieving aching feet, easing sprains, or stimulating the circulation for those prone to frostbite. The traditional mustard bath, using a heaping teaspoon of powdered mustard to a basin of hot water, is still an effective treatment today. Hot and cold treatments can also help reduce bruising and bring some relief for badly sprained ankles. Put the feet in a basin of very hot water containing a large handful of rosemary sprigs for 3–5 minutes and then plunge into a basin of iced water for 1–2 minutes. Repeat as many times as you can stand it.

EYEWASHES

EYEWASHES ARE SIMPLE to use and make, and can be very soothing for a range of eye complaints. The mixtures should not sting at all – if they do, dilute further, since individual sensitivity can vary. Use weak infusions or decoctions, or two drops of tincture to an eyecup filled with freshly boiled water. See the Caution right, about sterilizing the eyecup.

EQUIPMENT

• *Saucepan* • *Sieve* • *Jug* • *Eyecup*

STANDARD QUANTITY

Use 400 ml decoction, made with 15 g dried herb and 600 ml water (see p. 66), or 400 ml infusion, made with 15 g dried herb and 500 ml water (see p. 64), or 2 drops of tincture in an eyecup of freshly boiled water.

STANDARD APPLICATION

Bathe the eyes 3 times a day.

STORAGE

Store in a covered jug in a cool place. Make a fresh eyewash each day.

This eyewash is made with a decoction of pot marigold (Calendula officinalis) and eyebright (Euphrasia officinalis).

1 Make a decoction or infusion of your chosen herb. Simmer for 10–15 minutes to ensure sterility.

2 Strain well through a fine sieve. Make sure there are no particles of herb remaining that might irritate the eye.

3 Allow the mixture to cool to a lukewarm temperature and then fill an eyecup with the mixture.

4 Placing the eyecup over the eye, lean back so the eye is well wetted and blink several times.

GARGLES & MOUTHWASHES

GARGLES AND MOUTHWASHES can be made either from standard infusions and decoctions (to make, see pp. 64–67) or by diluting tinctures (to make, see p. 68). If using standard infusions or decoctions, strain well, allow the mixture to cool, and use in wineglass doses. If using tinctures, dilute 5 ml of tincture in a wineglass of warm water. Herbs will keep on working as they are digested, so gargles and mouthwashes made in this way can be swallowed as standard infusions and tinctures would be.

OVER-THE-COUNTER REMEDIES

THE DAYS WHEN HERBAL REMEDIES were only made at home are over. Today, the market in over-the-counter herbal products is huge, but choosing the right remedy is not always easy. In many countries products are carefully regulated: in Europe, for example, herbal remedies are licensed and their efficacy must be proven before medical claims can be made for them. For legal reasons, however, many remedies are not labeled with recommended medical uses, although their names may be suitably suggestive. If products and their actions are not clearly labeled, consumers should check the actions of individual herbs listed on the package. Where possible, it is always best to buy remedies from reputable suppliers with product licenses or to choose products on the recommendation of professional herbalists. Where it is given, consumers should follow the recommended dosage; otherwise, check the dosage with a professional herbalist.

Tablets & capsules

Herbs are usually sold in easy-to-take tablets or capsules. Most suppliers will provide information and sell plant mixes recommended for self-limiting ailments. A list of herbs commonly found in tablets and capsules follows:

BLUE FLAG – *for minor skin problems.*
BOLDO – *a digestive stimulant and urinary antiseptic sometimes sold in remedies for cystitis.*
BORAGE OIL, OR STAR FLOWER OIL – *rich in gamma-linolenic acid; sold as a supplement for menstrual disorders and skin complaints.*

BURDOCK – *mild laxtive action; promoted as a "spring cleaning" remedy.*
CASCARA – *a laxative; avoid when pregnant.*
CHASTEBERRY, OR AGNUS CASTUS – *usually recommended for various gynecological problems; overdose can cause formication (a sensation of ants crawling on the skin).*
CRANESBILL – *an astringent herb often used in commercial diarrhea remedies.*
DAMIANA – *sold as a general tonic and sometimes as an aphrodisiac.*
DANG GUI, OR TANG KWAI – *included as a tonic in specific women's remedies.*
DEVIL'S CLAW – *recommended for arthritis.*
ECHINACEA – *an immune stimulant for colds.*

EPHEDRA, OR MA HUANG – *often contained in patent sinusitis and cold remedies.*
EVENING PRIMROSE OIL – *rich in gamma-linolenic acid and marketed as a supplement for menstrual disorders and skin complaints.*
FENUGREEK – *used in digestive stimulants and milk stimulants for breastfeeding mothers.*
FEVERFEW – *for migraines and rheumatism.*
GARLIC – *used both as a cold cure and to help reduce cholesterol levels.*
GINGER –*used in motion sickness remedies.*
GINKGO – *a remedy for poor circulation.*
GINSENG – *a general purpose tonic.*
GOLDENSEAL – *a liver stimulant and de-congestant, often sold as an indigestion remedy.*

TABLETS & CAPSULES
Tablets are sold in a variety of bottles and packs.

Powders and oils in capsules.

Note: *For more information on herbs listed on these pages, see pp. 30–47 & pp. 138–40.*

OILS

Dropper

Dropper bottle

GOTU KOLA – *a tonic used in convalescence.*
GUARANA – *an all-purpose tonic.*
HELONIAS – *included in remedies for menstrual and menopausal problems.*
HE SHOU WU, OR FO TI – *a Chinese tonic herb used in some Western laxative mixtures but best regarded as a kidney tonic.*
HUANG QI, OR ASTRALAGUS ROOT – *a popular Chinese tonic.*
KELP – *a metabolic stimulant.*
PAPAYA – *a digestive remedy.*
PARSLEY – *often included in diuretic mixtures for premenstrual fluid retention.*
PILEWORT – *sometimes sold for internal consumption for hemorrhoids.*
PSYLLIUM SEEDS, OR ISPHAGULA – *laxative.*
SENNA – *laxative; avoid in pregnancy.*
SLIPPERY ELM – *for digestive problems and sore throats.*
UVA-URSI – *used in many diuretic mixtures for premenstrual fluid retention.*
VALERIAN – *used in calming mixtures for insomnia or nervous tension.*

Oils

When buying essential oils, choose well-known, reputable brands since oils are prone to adulteration and synthetic substitution. Quality products will be more expensive. Check effects in a specialist aromatherapy guide, and do not take essential oils internally except under professional direction.

Ointments & creams

Commercially available herbal ointments and creams tend to be limited to the most popular remedies. They may also be bought from suppliers of homeopathic and NewAge medicines under a variety of brand names. The following are commonly available:

ALOE VERA – *sold in cosmetic preparations but also valuable for sunburn and sores.*
ARNICA – *excellent for bruises and injuries but should not be used on broken skin.*
CHICKWEED – *draws infections from wounds and eases irritant skin conditions.*
COMFREY – *a restricted herb in many countries but a valuable and safe remedy when used externally for bruises and strains.*
CALENDULA OR POT MARIGOLD – *a useful antiseptic and antifungal, helpful for dry skin conditions.*
HYPERICUM OR ST.-JOHN'S-WORT – *often sold in combination with calendula for minor skin problems and burns.*
SAGE – *used for insect bites and as an all-purpose skin remedy.*
TEA TREE – *a potent antibacterial for scratches and skin infections.*
URTICA, OR STINGING NETTLE – *usually available from homeopathic suppliers for irritant skin conditions.*

Syrups, extracts & juices

Availability of liquid herbal extracts varies markedly between countries. In Germany, for example, a huge variety is available for professional use, sold by prescription, while in the US the range is more limited. Juices are sometimes for sale in health food stores and can be taken singly or combined with tinctures or syrups. Few products give any details of the herbs' action, so look them up before taking. Among the more useful juices that may be found are:

ARTICHOKE – *a liver stimulant and digestive remedy.*
BORAGE – *useful to stimulate adrenal glands and also used externally for irritating rashes on the skin.*
BLACK RADISH – *a digestive remedy.*
HORSETAIL – *rich in silica and suitable for deep-seated lung problems.*
OATS – *a tonic nervine useful for depression.*
RAMPS, OR WILD GARLIC – *a milder form of the familiar herb used in a similar way – to combat colds and help the immune system.*
SILVERWEED – *a decongestant member of the rose family that can be helpful for sinus problems.*

Oil in capsules
Oil bottle
OINTMENTS & CREAMS
Tubes of ointment
Pots of cream
SYRUPS, EXTRACTS & JUICES
Measuring spoon
Dark glass bottles are frequently used for storing syrups and other herbal remedies.

REMEDIES
❖ for ❖
COMMON
AILMENTS

DESPITE THE IMPORTANCE of pharmaceutical drugs, herbal remedies are still the most commonly used worldwide and in some countries they are the only medicines available. Herbal remedies provide safe, economical, and effective alternatives to orthodox medicines to treat a wide range of minor ills, and in our highly stressed world, the relaxing process of making a herbal infusion or preparing an ointment can be therapeutic in itself. Full instructions are given for the preparation of the remedies, but more detail can be found on pp. 62–79.

Essential Information

TREATMENT & DOSAGE

The remedies described in this book are safe, but overdose can be harmful. Do not exceed the suggested dose. Doubling the recommended quantity will not make the medicine twice as effective.

All recipes and dosages are for adults. Reduce the adult dose for children by following the guidelines on p. 128. The elderly may require lower doses than adults in their prime, due to a slower metabolism. Reduce doses by half for the very elderly or frail. Some herbs should not be used in pregnancy – see p. 126. Before taking a herbal remedy check any precautions (see pp. 30–47 and pp. 138–40).

The main remedy and supplementary treatments for each ailment may be taken individually or in combination. Unless otherwise stated, they should generally be used for 4–6 weeks. If there is no improvement, seek professional help. Some herbs interact with orthodox drugs; if you are already taking medication, consult a professional practitioner before taking home remedies. Do not suddenly stop taking medication without professional advice.

When several parts of a plant are available commercially, the particular component for a remedy (flower, root, etc.) is specified. **Essential oils** Do not take internally except under professional guidance. Dilute with a carrier oil before using externally.

VITAMIN & MINERAL SUPPLEMENTS

Specific recommendations for the use of supplements to treat particular ailments are made throughout. If taking supplements for general health, opt for a multivitamin or multimineral preparation to prevent imbalance. Select reputable brands and consult a medical practitioner over any long-term use (i.e., more then 2–3 months). Do not exceed the recommended dose on the package. Excessive intake of mineral supplements can be damaging. When taken in excess, the water-soluble vitamins (B and C) are generally excreted, but the fat-soluble group (A, D, E, and K) can damage the liver. Do not take fat-soluble vitamin supplements for more than 3–4 weeks without professional advice. Daily recommended doses vary enormously, but in general do not exceed the following:

VITAMIN A – *10,000 IUs daily for children, in pregnancy and for those seeking to become pregnant. 20,000 IUs daily for other adults.*
VITAMIN B6 – *50 mg daily.*
VITAMIN D – *400 IUs daily.*
VITAMIN E – *600 IUs daily. If taking blood-thinning medication do not take vitamin E except under close medical supervision.*

Abbreviations:
IU International Unit. The potency of vitamins is sometimes measured in IUs. Their equivalent in grams varies according to the mixture used in the product.
mg milligram (one-thousandth of a gram).
µg microgram (one-millionth of a gram).

COUGHS & COLDS

CONVENTIONAL AND HERBAL medicine argue that when stress builds up, opportunist bacteria and viruses move in, causing coughs, colds, and flu, although some psychologists reason that these ailments provide the chance to take a much-needed rest from day-to day responsibilities. Such ailments should not be left untreated, since colds, for example, can easily turn into more serious disorders, or leave lingering coughs and persistent phlegm. Early treatment is the answer.

Chest coughs

The act of coughing removes irritant particles from the airways. Chest coughs are loose and produce white, yellow, or green phlegm. Colored phlegm may indicate an infection or bronchitis.

THYME & LUNGWORT SYRUP

This soothing expectorant mixture is made with thyme, a useful antiseptic for the respiratory system, and lungwort leaves, which were once said to resemble diseased lungs, hence the plant's use for chest infections.

~ INGREDIENTS ~
10 g licorice juice stick (*Glycyrrhiza glabra*)
750 ml water
10 g dried thyme (*Thymus vulgaris*)
10 g dried lungwort leaves (*Pulmonaria officinalis*)
5 g dried cowslip flowers (*Primula veris*)
5 g anise seeds (*Pimpinella anisum*)
500 g honey

~ HOW TO MAKE THE SYRUP ~

1 Put the licorice and water in a pan and heat until the licorice has dissolved.

2 Mix the herbs and the seeds together and pour on the hot licorice juice. Steep for 10 minutes and strain.

3 Return the strained mixture, which should amount to about 500 ml, to the pan and add the honey. Heat the mixture gently until simmering and stir constantly until the honey is dissolved. Allow the mixture to cool, pour into sterilized, dark glass bottles, and seal with cork stoppers.

DOSAGE *Take a 5 ml dose up to 6 times a day while symptoms persist.*

LICORICE *is a soothing expectorant, ideal for stubborn coughs. It also helps to flavor the mixture and make it palatable.*

Licorice juice sticks

COWSLIP *is rich in saponins, which have an expectorant effect.*

Fresh cowslip flowers

Dried cowslip flowers

Fresh thyme

THYME *is a good antiseptic for chest infections.*

Dried thyme leaves

LUNGWORT *contains allantoin, a healing chemical that helps to repair damage to the mucous lining of the airways. It is also an effective expectorant.*

Fresh lungwort

Dried lungwort leaves

Anise seeds

ANISE *is an expectorant and antispasmodic. It gives the syrup a pleasant flavor.*

HONEY *preserves the herbs and is particularly soothing. Its sweetness flavors the cough mixture.*

Honey

SUPPLEMENTARY TREATMENTS

■ Supplement the cough syrup with a chest rub made by adding 2–3 drops each of eucalyptus, marjoram, and thyme essential oils to 10 ml sweet almond or wheat germ oil. Massage a little on to the chest 3–4 times a day.

■ Take 2–3 x 200 mg echinacea capsules 3 times a day or 5–10 ml of echinacea tincture (to make, see p. 68) in 100 ml warm water up to 4 times a day to combat infection.

CAUTIONS FOR COUGHS

• *Persistent or recurrent coughs at any age can be a sign of more serious health problems. Seek professional help if the cough lasts for more than a week or so, if there is chest pain, or if there is no obviously associated cold or infection.*

• *If the phlegm from a productive cough is streaked with blood, or if the infection is slow to clear, seek professional help.*

Thyme & lungwort syrup

THYME & LUNGWORT SYRUP soothes and relieves chest coughs. Homemade syrups can be stored in sterile bottles for several months. It is important to use a cork stopper, since syrups often ferment, and screw-topped bottles may explode.

Irritant coughs

Irritating, dry, or "unproductive" coughs can be debilitating. They are often associated with nervous tension and anxiety, rather than infections, and may respond to soothing cough suppressants.

WILD CHERRY & HYSSOP SYRUP

Wild cherry is a mild sedative, good for suppressing irritable or racking coughs, or when further coughing is exhausting and unhelpful. It is combined with hyssop, a traditional remedy for stubborn coughs.

~ INGREDIENTS ~
30 g dried wild cherry bark (*Prunus serotina*)
250 ml & 100 ml water
10 g dried hyssop (*Hyssopus officinalis*)
250 g honey

~ HOW TO MAKE THE SYRUP ~

1 Soak the cherry bark in 250 ml water overnight. Strain the liquid and reduce slightly by simmering gently for 15 minutes to make a decoction.

2 Meanwhile, make a standard infusion of the hyssop in 100 ml water (see p. 64), strain, and add the liquid to the reduced bark decoction.

3 Add the honey and simmer for 5–10 minutes to produce a syrup. Allow the mixture to cool and store in sterilized, dark glass bottles with cork stoppers.

DOSAGE *Take 5 ml up to 4 times a day while symptoms persist.*

Note: See CAUTIONS FOR COUGHS *on p. 85.*

Wild cherry & hyssop syrup

Dried wild cherry bark

Common colds

The common cold is caused by viral infection and is usually characterized by the familiar dry throat and running nose, in some cases progressing to feverishness and persistent coughs.

BONESET & ELDERFLOWER TEA

Boneset was used in North America for bone-shaking fevers, not for treating fractures as its name may suggest. Elderflower is added to combat phlegm.

~ INGREDIENTS ~
10g dried boneset (*Eupatorium perfoliatum*)
10g dried elderflower (*Sambucus nigra*)
5g dried yarrow (*Achillea millefolium*)
5g dried peppermint (*Mentha piperita*)
500 ml water

~ HOW TO MAKE THE TEA ~

Mix the herbs in a teapot and pour on freshly boiled water. Steep for 10 minutes and strain into a jug. Cover, and store in a cool place.

DOSAGE *Take a wineglass dose every 3–4 hours as long as symptoms persist. Flavor with honey if desired.*

Supplementary treatments
■ If you feel shivery and chilled, drink a warming decoction of ginger and other spicy herbs to encourage sweating. Try the recipe for Ginger & Cinnamon Tea on p. 108.
■ Take immune stimulants to fight the infection: echinacea – 100 mg tablets up to 4 times daily, or 5 ml of tincture up to 4 times daily; or garlic – 2 x 200 mg capsules 3 times a day.
■ Eat plenty of fruit and avoid mucus-forming foods, such as dairy products, refined carbohydrates, and alcohol.

Fresh hyssop

Flu

We often describe a bad cold as "flu," but the real thing can also include fever, coughing, head and body pains, nausea, and vomiting. It often leaves the sufferer feeling debilitated and depressed for several weeks afterward.

—— *ELECAMPANE & VERVAIN MIXTURE* ——

Elecampane is an excellent tonic expectorant and restorative, while vervain encourages sweating to help reduce fevers and aids the digestion.

~ INGREDIENTS ~

10g dried elecampane root (*Inula helenium*)
5g dried pleurisy root (*Asclepias tuberosa*)
5g dried vervain (*Verbena officinalis*)
5g dried licorice root (*Glycyrrhiza glabra*)
5g dried boneset (*Eupatorium perfoliatum*)
500 ml water

~ HOW TO MAKE THE MIXTURE ~

1 Heat the elecampane and pleurisy root in the water. Simmer gently for 15 minutes to make a decoction. Meanwhile, mix the other herbs in a teapot or lidded jug.

2 Pour the simmering decoction over the dried herbs. Steep for 10 minutes and strain. Store in a cool place.

DOSAGE *Take a wineglass dose 3 times a day. Continue taking the mixture for a couple of weeks after the attack as a tonic.*

Supplementary treatments

■ Take the teas described for colds and fevers as necessary.
■ Take 3 x 200 mg echinacea capsules 3 times a day (to make the capsules, see p. 70).
■ Use a compress (to make, see p. 71) soaked in lavender infusion to ease feverish headaches.
■ Drink a standard infusion of St.-John's-wort and lemon balm tea (to make, see p. 64) if depression is a problem.

Fevers

High temperature is part of the body's normal response to infection. Traditional fever management is aimed at helping the body fight infection by either cooling with herbs to encourage sweating, or maintaining body temperature with heating remedies.

CAUTION

• *Professional support is needed for high fevers – seek medical help if body temperatures rise over 102°F (39°C).*

—— *CATNIP & VERVAIN TEA* ——

This is a cooling mixture for use when the fever is at the hot, sticky stage. Catnip is a sedative herb that encourages sweating, and vervain is a good digestive stimulant.

~ INGREDIENTS ~

40 g dried catnip (*Nepeta cataria*)
30 g dried vervain (*Verbena officinalis*)
30 g dried boneset (*Eupatorium perfoliatum*)
water

~ HOW TO MAKE THE TEA ~

1 Mix the herbs and store in a dry, airtight container.

2 Put 2–3 teaspoonfuls of the mix in a tisane cup or small teapot. Add a cup of freshly boiled water and steep for 10 minutes. Strain.

DOSAGE *Sip a cup of the mixture as often as possible until body temperature drops.*

Supplementary treatments

■ During the chill stages of a fever drink a warming tea. Try the Ginger & Cinnamon Tea given on p. 108.
■ Take 5–10 ml of echinacea tincture 3 times a day to combat infections (to make, see p. 68).

OVER-THE-COUNTER REMEDIES Coughs & Colds

■ Patent cough and cold remedies are readily available, containing herbs such as astragalus (*Huang Qi*), aniseed, bloodroot, boneset, cowslip, cloves, echinacea, eucalyptus, fennel, hyssop, ipecacuanha, licorice, peppermint, and sundew.
■ Over-the-counter inhalants can help congestion. They usually contain cajeput, clove, eucalyptus, peppermint, and juniper oils, and sometimes added menthol, an active ingredient of peppermint oil.
■ Use elderflower and peppermint teabags together, as a quick option for minor colds. Alternatively, dilute elderflower cordial with hot water and sip.

EARS, NOSE & THROAT

THE MUCOUS MEMBRANES of the nose and throat are the body's first line of defense in keeping dust and toxins out of the system and away from the lungs. Microscopic hair cells constantly beat stray particles out of the way and move them down toward the stomach. These defenses have to work overtime in our polluted environment and it is not surprising that sometimes they fail, paving the way for disorders of the nose, throat, and ears.

Note: Ears, nose, and throat problems can be related to various other disorders. See also coughs & colds pp. 84–6; hay fever p. 100; sinus headaches p. 110.

Sore throats & laryngitis

Sore throats often herald the onset of colds and flu, or they can be a symptom of overworked vocal chords. They may also signal local inflammation and infection as with laryngitis and pharyngitis – inflammations of the vocal chords or nasal cavities.

SAGE & ROSEMARY GARGLE

One of the best combinations for sore throats and laryngitis: both rosemary and sage are aromatic, antiseptic, and rich in potent healing oils. Additional astringents, such as lady's mantle, can also help reduce inflammation.

~ INGREDIENTS ~

15 g dried, or 45 g fresh purple sage leaves
(*Salvia officinalis* 'Purpurea')
10 g dried, or 20 g fresh rosemary leaves
(*Rosmarinus officinalis*)
5 g dried lady's mantle leaves (*Alchemilla vulgaris*)
500 ml water

~ HOW TO MAKE THE GARGLE ~

1 Mix the herbs together in a teapot or jug and add freshly boiled water.

2 Steep for 10 minutes, strain, and allow the mixture to cool. Cover and store in a cool place.

DOSAGE *Gargle with a wineglassful at a time every 2–3 hours while symptoms persist. The tea is antiseptic and healing, so swallow the mixture after gargling.*

Supplementary treatments

■ Add 5 ml of echinacea tincture (to make, see p. 68) to each gargle or take separately to combat infections. Take 2 x 200 mg capsules of dried, powdered garlic 3 times a day to support the immune system.

■ Laryngitis and pharyngitis can be helped by steam inhalations: add 2 drops each of sandalwood, lavender, and frankincense essential oils to a bowl of boiling water and inhale the steam for 10 minutes (see p. 78). Stay in a warm room for at least 30 minutes afterward.

■ Add the same oils to 5 ml of sweet almond oil and massage the mixture around the throat.

Sage & rosemary gargle

Lady's mantle

Sage

Rosemary

Tonsillitis

The tonsils, found at the back of the throat, are a type of lymph gland, part of the body's immune system. Persistent infection can signify weakened immunity or constant underlying physical stress, such as food intolerance or exhaustion. Cutting out potential irritant foods, such as milk or wheat, may help; so can a good relaxing vacation.

—— CLEAVERS & SAGE TINCTURE ——

Cleavers is cleansing and healing for the lymphatic system. In this remedy it is combined with sage, an antiseptic, and other antibacterials and immune stimulants, to help combat tonsillitis.

~ INGREDIENTS ~
50 ml cleavers tincture (*Galium aparine*)
15 ml sage tincture (*Salvia officinalis*)
25 ml echinacea tincture (*Echinacea angustifolia*)
10 ml goldenseal tincture (*Hydrastis canadensis*)

~ HOW TO MAKE THE TINCTURE ~
1 To make the individual tinctures, see p. 68.

2 Combine all the tinctures in a sterilized, dark glass bottle and mix well.

DOSAGE *Take 10 ml of the mixture in half a tumbler of hot water 3 times a day during the acute stage; adding a little honey if desired. Reduce to 5 ml in hot water 3 times a day, as symptoms ease.*

CAUTIONS
• *Abscesses on the tonsils (quinsy) need professional help.*
• *Seek help if there is fever, especially in children.*

Supplementary treatments
■ Use the gargle on p. 88 for sore throats, substituting thyme leaves for rosemary, as they are more antiseptic.
■ Strengthen the immune system by taking either 1 g vitamin C, 2 x 200 mg capsules of dried, powdered garlic 3 times a day, or 2–3 x 200 mg *Astragalus/Huang Qi* capsules daily for a few weeks to prevent further attacks.
■ Drink a soothing infusion daily made with 10 g each of dried ground ivy, pot marigold petals and chamomile flowers (to make, see p. 64).
■ Add 5 drops each of thyme, and marjoram essential oils and a single drop of rose oil to 25 ml of sweet almond oil and massage into the neck area. Use the same mix of oils in a steam inhalation (to use, see p. 78).

Mouth ulcers

Painful ulcers in the mouth – known as aphthae – are often related to opportunist fungal or bacterial infections gaining a hold when sufferers are exhausted and run down. Sometimes ulcers are associated with excessive sugar consumption, which fuels fungal growths. They can also be linked to stomach upsets.

—— MYRRH & ROSEMARY MOUTHWASH ——

Myrrh is extremely antimicrobial. It is one of the less pleasant-tasting herbs, however, and rosemary infusion is added to help disguise the flavor.

~ INGREDIENTS ~
30 g dried rosemary (*Rosmarinus officinalis*)
15 ml myrrh tincture or 5 drops myrrh oil (*Commiphora molmol*)
500 ml water

~ HOW TO MAKE THE MOUTHWASH ~
1 To make the tincture, see p. 68.

2 Put the rosemary in a jug or teapot and add freshly boiled water. Steep for 10 minutes and strain.

3 Add the myrrh tincture or myrrh oil to the rosemary infusion and stir well. Cover and store in a cool place.

DOSAGE *Use a wineglass of the mixture as a mouthwash every 4 hours until symptoms ease.*

Supplementary treatments
■ Chew bilberries after the mouthwash to help disguise the flavor and promote healing.
■ Apply a drop of clove oil directly to the mouth ulcer – this will probably sting, but it can be very effective.
■ Take 2 x 200 mg echinacea capsules 3 times a day to combat infection.
■ Persistent fungal infections may be the cause of mouth ulcers. Avoid sugary food and dairy products, eat plenty of garlic, and take pot marigold infusion (to make, see p. 64) as a daily tea.
■ Take professional advice if mouth ulcers are persistent or severe as they can be related to food intolerance. In particular, they commonly indicate sensitivity to gluten. They may also be a sign of iron deficiency, or of vitamins B_{12}, or B_6, or of folic acid.

Phlegm

The protective membranes lining the nasal passages produce mucus as a form of protection in response to infections or irritants. Excess mucus – phlegm – often follows a common cold. It is also caused by allergens, such as pollen and house dust.

——— SANDALWOOD & PINE INHALANT———

Steam inhalants are one of the most effective ways of treating upper respiratory tract problems. These oils are astringent, antiseptic, and soothing.

~ INGREDIENTS ~

15 drops sandalwood oil (*Santalum album*)
15 drops pine oil (*Pinus sylvestris*)
10 drops lavender oil (*Lavandula angustifolia*)
5 drops peppermint oil (*Mentha piperita*)
45 ml compound tincture of benzoin
– friar's balsam (*Styrax benzoin*)

~ HOW TO USE THE INHALANT ~

1 Mix the ingredients in a 50 ml sterilized, dark glass bottle and shake well.

2 Fill a basin with boiling water. Add a teaspoon of the mix to the water. Lean over the water and cover the head and basin with a towel. Inhale the steam for 10 minutes. Repeat twice a day while the condition persists.

Note: Stay in a warm room for at least 30 minutes afterward.

Supplementary treatments

■ Mix 30 ml each of eyebright, ribwort plantain, and echinacea tinctures with 10 ml of goldenseal tincture (to make, see p. 68). Sip a 5 ml dose diluted in warm water 3 times a day.
■ Take 2 x 200 mg garlic capsules 3 times a day.

Peppermint

Sandalwood & pine inhalant

Pine

Sinusitis

The sinuses are cavities in the skull. They can be prone to inflammation and overproduction of mucus, leading to headaches, gum pains, and watery eyes. Learning to relax and manage stress has a marked effect on sinusitis, and the condition often responds to the action of warming herbs.

— MAGNOLIA & ELDERFLOWER TINCTURE —

Magnolia is an excellent anti-inflammatory for the mucous membranes, and elderflower is a traditional remedy for congestion and phlegm.

~ INGREDIENTS ~

25 ml magnolia flower tincture
(*Xin Yi Hua/Magnolia liliflora*)
25 ml elderflower tincture (*Sambucus nigra*)
15 ml ground ivy tincture (*Glechoma hederacea*)
15 ml echinacea tincture (*Echinacea angustifolia*)
10 ml bayberry tincture (*Myrica cerifera*)
5 ml ginger tincture (*Zingiber officinalis*)
5 ml peppermint tincture (*Mentha piperita*)

~ HOW TO MAKE THE TINCTURE ~

To make the individual tinctures, see p. 68. Combine them in a 100 ml sterilized, dark glass bottle and shake.

DOSAGE *Take 5 ml in half a tumbler of warm water 3 times a day before meals while symptoms persist.*

Supplementary treatments

■ Make a cream (see p. 76) by adding 10 ml bayberry tincture and 5 ml elderflower tincture (to make, see p. 68), to 50 ml melted emulsifying ointment (available over the counter). Apply the cream to the sinus areas 2 or 3 times a day, massaging gently.
■ Add 5 drops of sandalwood oil to a saucer of water on the bedside table to relieve symptoms at night.
■ Take 2 x 200 mg capsules of dried, powdered garlic 3 times a day and take extra vitamin C. A 24- or 48-hour fruit fast may help. (The weak or elderly should take professional advice before fasting.)
■ See p. 110 for advice on treating sinus headaches.

Lavender

Sandalwood

Earache

Earache may be caused by local acute infection, but can also be related to sinus problems, mumps, or toothache. Identifying the cause is important. Recurring ear infections, especially in children, can be associated with food intolerance (see p. 101).

CAUTIONS
- *Seek professional help if pain is severe, especially in children. Get help: if there is pain in the mastoid bone (behind the ear); if there is a discharge from the ear; or if the condition persists.*
- *Do not put anything into the ear if the eardrum is perforated; seek medical advice if unsure.*

— MULLEIN & PASQUE FLOWER EARDROPS —
Pasque flower is a good sedative and analgesic that seems to have a specific affinity with the ears, while mullein is a herb with soothing properties that helps repair damaged tissues.

·· INGREDIENTS ~
20 drops pasque flower tincture (*Anemone vulgaris*)
24 ml infused mullein oil (*Verbascum thapsus*)
20 drops goldenseal tincture (*Hydrastis canadensis*)

~ HOW TO MAKE THE EARDROPS ~
To make the tinctures and infused oil, see pp. 68 and 72. Mix the ingredients in a sterilized dropper bottle. Shake.

APPLICATION *Using the dropper, put 2 drops into the ear and cover with a cotton plug. Repeat 3 times a day.*

Supplementary treatments
■ Massage the mastoid bone (behind the ear), in front of the ear, and at the back of the neck with a mix of 2 ml each of lavender and tea tree oil in 20 ml of sweet almond oil to reduce the risk of infection spreading.
■ Take 2 x 200 mg capsules of dried powdered garlic 3 times daily and a zinc and vitamin C supplement.
■ Avoid mucous-forming foods such as dairy products.

Chronic ear infection

Inflammation of the middle ear (*otitis media*) is common at all ages. When it causes fluid to collect it can lead to deafness, and this condition is most common in children. In addition to progressive hearing loss, it is characterized by earache and copious sticky secretions. Some researchers have associated it with allergy to cow's milk. Orthodox treatment usually involves inserting tubes in the eardrum to relieve the build-up of fluid.

—— GOLDENROD & GINKGO MIXTURE ——
Goldenrod is a good decongestant that can be helpful in ear conditions, while both ginkgo and pasque flower have an affinity with ear problems, helping to focus healing mixtures on the ear. The doses given here are suitable for children aged 4–6, the most frequent sufferers. See p. 128 for general advice on children's dosage.

~ INGREDIENTS ~
40 ml goldenrod tincture (*Solidago virgaurea*)
25 ml ginkgo tincture (*Ginkgo biloba*)
15 ml ribwort plantain tincture (*Plantago lanceolata*)
10 ml St.-John's-wort tincture (*Hypericum perforatum*)
10 ml pasque flower tincture (*Anemone vulgaris*)

~ HOW TO MAKE THE MIXTURE ~
To make the individual tinctures see p. 68. Combine them in a 100 ml sterilized, dark glass bottle and shake well.

DOSAGE *Take 20 drops in a glass of fruit juice 3 times a day.*

Supplementary treatments
■ Take a 200 mg goldenseal capsule daily. Alternatively, add 5 ml of the goldenseal tincture to the main remedy and use a strongly flavored juice, such as black currant, to dilute the mixture, since goldenseal has a very bitter taste.
■ Replace cow's milk in the diet with soy products and reduce sugar intake as much as possible.

OVER-THE-COUNTER REMEDIES *Ears, Nose & Throat*

■ For congestive problems, look for capsules or tablets combining any of the following astringent, antiseptic, soothing herbs: agrimony, bayberry bark, cloves, elderflower, eucalyptus, eyebright, goldenrod, goldenseal, magnolia flowers, marshmallow, peppermint, white horehound, wild indigo, and yarrow.

■ Look for ready-mixed inhalants, such as those based on friar's balsam.
■ Try herbal nasal sprays that combine eucalyptus and peppermint oils.
■ Use herbal teabags containing elderflower, pot marigold, or peppermint to supplement other therapeutic approaches.

EYE COMPLAINTS

THE EYES ARE in constant use transmitting images, a task made much harder by having to cope with computer screens, the dust and grit of city streets, and sunlight that is becoming progressively brighter, due to ozone depletion. Regular exercises, such as alternately focusing on near and distant objects, can help hardworking eyes. Splashing them with cold water each morning can also help to keep them working well. Herbal remedies are very useful for soothing the symptoms of many common eye complaints.

GENERAL CAUTION
• *Eye infections can be very contagious – avoid sharing face towels or face cloths.*

Styes

A stye is an inflammation of the glands found at the base of the eyelashes. It is caused by a bacterial infection and is generally a sign that the sufferer is run down. Rest, relaxation, and a good diet are just as important as topical treatments.

———— MARIGOLD COMPRESS ————

Astringent and antiseptic, marigold is an excellent remedy for local skin infections and inflammations.

~ INGREDIENTS ~
25 g dried pot marigold petals (*Calendula officinalis*)
500 ml water

~ HOW TO MAKE THE COMPRESS ~

1 Pour freshly boiled water on to the pot marigold petals. Steep for 10 minutes and strain.

2 As soon as the infusion is cool enough to handle, soak a small square of muslin or other fabric in it.

APPLICATION *Wring out the fabric and apply it to the stye, holding it to the affected area until the compress cools. Repeat with a fresh compress at frequent intervals during the day, reheating the infusion as necessary, until the infection subsides. Make a fresh infusion daily.*

Supplementary treatments
■ Boost the immune system with or 2 x 200 mg echinacea capsules 3 times a day.
■ Drink an infusion 2 or 3 times a day made from equal parts of cleavers, *Ju Hua* (dried Chinese chrysanthemum flowers), fumitory, and burdock leaf. (To make, see p. 64.)

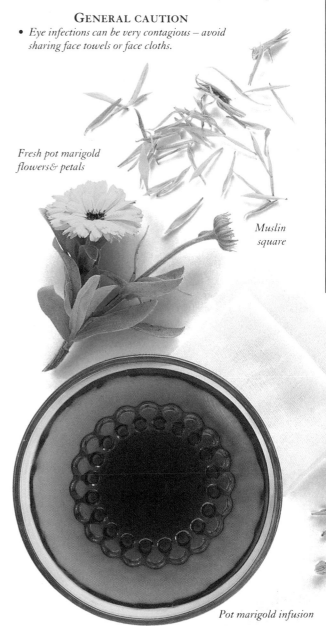

Fresh pot marigold flowers & petals

Muslin square

Pot marigold infusion

Conjunctivitis & blepharitis

Conjunctivitis, commonly known as "pink eye," is an inflammation of the mucous membrane covering the eyeball. Blepharitis is inflammation of the eyelid. Both are usually caused by infection, although conjunctivitis can also be associated with dusty air, or a drying of the eye's normal secretions in old age.

—— EYEBRIGHT & MARIGOLD EYEWASH ——

Eyebright, as its name suggests, is a herb traditionally used to treat infections. It is a tiny, semiparasitic plant found in grass meadows and rarely grown in herb gardens.

~ INGREDIENTS ~

15 g dried eyebright (*Euphrasia officinalis*)
10 g dried pot marigold petals (*Calendula officinalis*)
500 ml water

~ HOW TO MAKE THE EYEWASH ~

[1] Mix the herbs and water together and heat in a pan.

[2] Simmer for 5–10 minutes to sterilize the herbs. Strain, and allow to cool completely. Store in a sterilized bottle.

APPLICATION *Pour a little into a sterilized eyecup and bathe the eye thoroughly. If both eyes are affected, sterilize the eyecup again and pour a fresh amount of the mixture into the eyecup, before bathing the other eye. Repeat frequently in acute cases. Make a fresh mixture each day. Note. See p. 62 for instructions on sterilizing*

CAUTION

• *Seek professional help if the infection does not resolve within a day or so, or if there is decreased vision or pain in the eye.*

Supplementary treatments

■ Apply cold, used teabags of Indian, Chinese, or fennel tea to the eyes as poultices, and relax for 15 minutes.
■ To combat infection, drink a standard infusion of eyebright 3 times a day (to make, see p. 64), and take 2 x 200 mg echinacea capsules 3 times a day while symptoms persist.

Tired eyes & eye strain

Stress, long working hours, and pollution all combine to make eye strain a common problem. The simple answer is to take regular breaks from computer screens, avoid working all day in artificial light, frequently focus on distant objects for a few seconds as a break from close work, or close the eyes and press very gently on the eyelids with the palms.

—— JU HUA & WOOD BETONY TEA ——

In Chinese medicine the eyes are associated with the liver, and herbs such as Ju Hua *and wood betony, which clean and stimulate that organ, can help revive the eyes.*

~ INGREDIENTS ~

25 g *Ju Hua* (dried, prepared Chinese chrysanthemum flowers – *Chrysanthemum morifolium*)
20 g dried wood betony (*Stachys betonia*)
10 g dried *gotu kola* (*Centella asiatica*)
5 g dried peppermint (*Mentha piperita*)
water

~ HOW TO MAKE THE TEA ~

[1] Mix the herbs and store in a dark, airtight container.

[2] Put 2–3 teaspoons of the mix in a tisane cup or small teapot. Add a cup of freshly boiled water and steep for 10 minutes. Strain.

DOSAGE *Take a break from work and drink a cup when the eyes feel tired.*

Supplementary treatments

■ Place slices of fresh cucumber on each closed eye and relax for 10–15 minutes.
■ Take 1–2 g vitamin C and 10,000–20,000 IUs vitamin A (except in pregnancy).
■ Bathe eyes with Eyebright & Marigold Eyewash (left) or with 5 drops of self-heal tincture (to make, see p. 68) in an eyecup of warm water.

OVER-THE-COUNTER REMEDIES *Eye Complaints*

Fresh pot marigold

■ Apply a tiny dab of ready made calendula cream directly to styes.
■ Use store-bought elderflower, fennel, pot marigold, or raspberry leaf teabags to make an infusion. Allow to cool and then apply them to inflamed and tired eyes as a cold poultice to relieve symptoms.

SKIN & HAIR PROBLEMS

THE SKIN FORMS a remarkable defensive barrier against the outside world. It harbors a thriving community of bacteria to ward off unfriendly micro-organisms and contains millions of sensory nerve endings. Its efficiency is a good guide to our general health and well-being, and herbal remedies for skin complaints usually focus on internal medication to restore a healthy balance in the body.

Dried heartsease aerial parts

Fresh heartsease

HEARTSEASE *contains saponins, which are very cleansing. It also relieves inflamed tissues and strengthens blood vessels.*

Eczema

Irritant skin inflammation may be due to allergy to foods (see p. 101) or contact with particular chemicals, and can often become worse with stress. Calming remedies can help to reduce attacks, and cleansing herbs remove toxins from the system.

Fresh clover

—HEARTSEASE & RED CLOVER TEA—

Heartsease is a good cleansing and anti-inflammatory herb, which also acts as a gentle circulatory stimulant. Red clover also helps clear toxins from the system and has a diuretic action.

Dried clover flowers

RED CLOVER *is an anti-inflammatory and cleansing herb for skin problems.*

~ INGREDIENTS ~
20 g dried heartsease (*Viola tricolor*)
20 g dried red clover flowers (*Trifolium pratense*)
20 g dried stinging nettle (*Urtica dioica*)
20 g dried burdock (*Arctium lappa*)
10 g dried skullcap (*Scutellaria lateriflora*)
10 g dried fumitory (*Fumaria officinalis*)
500 ml water

Fresh nettles

Crushed dried nettle

~ HOW TO MAKE THE TEA ~

1 Mix the herbs and store in an airtight jar. Spoon 25 g of the mixture into a teapot.

2 Pour 500 ml of freshly boiled water on to the mixture. Steep for 10 minutes and strain. Cover and store the surplus in a cool place.

DOSAGE *Take a wineglass dose 3 times a day before meals. (See p. 83 for advice on length of treatment.)*

STINGING NETTLE *is rich in vitamins and minerals and stimulates the circulation.*

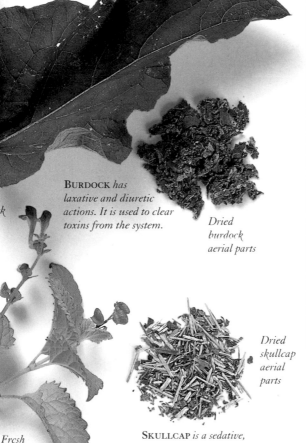

Fresh burdock

BURDOCK *has laxative and diuretic actions. It is used to clear toxins from the system.*

Dried burdock aerial parts

Fresh skullcap

Dried skullcap aerial parts

SKULLCAP *is a sedative, enabling the system to cope with the stress that often exacerbates eczema.*

FUMITORY *helps to stimulate the digestion and has a cleansing action.*

Fresh fumitory

Dried fumitory aerial parts

Heartsease & red clover tea

SUPPLEMENTARY TREATMENTS

■ Use pot marigold or chamomile creams externally for dry eczema. Try chickweed cream to reduce itching. To make creams, see p. 76.

■ For oozing eczema make a standard infusion (to make, see p. 64) of heartsease and pot marigold petals. Strain, allow to cool, and soak a compress in the mixture. Apply to the affected part.

■ Evening primrose oil can help in some types of eczema: take 2 x 1 g capsules daily. Make sure an adequate supply of vitamins A, B, C, and E are in the diet, as well as magnesium, zinc, and calcium. Take supplements if necessary.

■ Relieve itching with a lotion made from 35 ml each of borage juice, distilled witch hazel, and rosewater. Apply frequently with a cotton ball.

HEARTSEASE & RED CLOVER TEA relieves eczema by cleansing the system of toxins, calming the nerves and soothing inflammation.

Psoriasis

Psoriasis involves overproduction of certain skin cells, which causes patches of silvery scaling usually found on the knees, elbows, or scalp. It is quite common in the West and in rare cases it can become very severe, affecting large parts of the body and may be associated with chronic rheumatic disorders.

——— FIGWORT TEA ———

Psoriasis is an ailment that seems to come and go, and is often helped by sunshine and seawater. Cleansing, anti-inflammatory herbs, such as figwort and red clover, can also help.

~ INGREDIENTS ~
10 g fresh burdock root (*Arctium lappa*)
5 g fresh yellow dock root (*Rumex crispus*)
15 g fresh figwort (*Scrophularia nodosa*)
10 g fresh red clover flowers (*Trifolium pratense*)
750 ml water

~ HOW TO MAKE THE TEA ~

[1] Mix the burdock and yellow dock together in a saucepan and add the water. Bring to the boil and simmer for 15 minutes, to make a concentrate.

[2] Put the figwort and red clover flowers together in a teapot or jug. Pour the burdock and yellow dock concentrate over these herbs and steep for 10 minutes. Strain. Store in a covered jug.

DOSAGE *Take a wineglass dose 3 times a day. See p. 83 for advice on how long to take. Flavor with honey or lemon juice as required.*

Supplementary treatments
■ Cleavers cream (to make, see p. 76) can be useful for treating small patches or the early stages of psoriasis. Apply 2 or 3 times a day to affected areas.
■ If the scalp is affected, make a hair rinse using 10 ml of rosemary tincture (to make, see p. 68) and 10 drops of juniper oil in 500 ml of warm water. Apply after shampooing as a final rinse.
■ Psoriasis often seems to go with a tense, insular personality. Bach Flower Remedies such as crab apple, agrimony, willow, or water violet can sometimes help.
■ Avoid alcohol and herbs such as yarrow, cinnamon twigs, and linden flowers, as these increase peripheral circulation and stimulate the skin.
■ Take 1 g vitamin C and 1–2 g kelp tablets daily, as well as zinc and vitamin A (follow the instructions on the package).

Urticaria (hives)

Urticaria and hives are names for a rash of red itchy lumps and blisters on the skin. They can be caused by contact with irritant allergens, such as those found in plants like stinging nettles, hops, runner beans, or borage. Chemicals such as salicylates, found in aspirin and in many foods, can have a similar effect, causing rashes that most often occur around the mouth.

——— AGRIMONY & CHAMOMILE TEA ———

Persistent urticaria is generally related to food allergies. This soothing infusion contains agrimony, a useful herb for calming gut irritations, and chamomile, which has antiallergenic properties.

~ INGREDIENTS ~
10 g dried agrimony (*Agrimonia eupatoria*)
10 g dried chamomile flowers (*Matricaria recutita*)
5 g dried stinging nettles (*Urtica dioica*)
5 g dried heartsease (*Viola tricolor*)
500 ml water

~ HOW TO MAKE THE TEA ~

Mix all the dried herbs together and add freshly boiled water. Steep for 5 minutes and strain into a jug. Cover and store in a cool place.

DOSAGE *Take a wineglass dose 3 times a day until the rash subsides.*

Supplementary treatments
■ Rub the area with sliced onion or crushed cabbage leaves.
■ Use chamomile cream (available over the counter – to make, see p. 76) on affected areas several times a day.
■ If stress is a contributory factor, drink an infusion of skullcap (to make, see p. 64) 3 times a day.

Agrimony & chamomile tea

Chamomile

Agrimony

Tea tree oil

Infused pot marigold oil

Pot marigold

Marigold & tea tree ointment

Ringworm & athlete's foot

Skin infections, like ringworm and athlete's foot, are often caused by common fungi, which attack when the immune system is weakened by stress or exhaustion. Fungi thrive in damp, confined conditions, for example between poorly washed or dried toes.

— MARIGOLD & TEA TREE OINTMENT —

Both pot marigold and tea tree are extremely antifungal. Using an ointment helps to keep the affected areas dry, which discourages the fungi. Combining the two oils for use as a lotion is a convenient alternative.

~ INGREDIENTS ~
25 ml infused pot marigold oil (*Calendula officinalis*)
8 g beeswax
8 g anhydrous lanolin
5 ml tea tree oil (*Melaleuca alternifolia*)

~ HOW TO MAKE THE OINTMENT ~

1 To make the infused pot marigold oil, see p. 73.

2 Melt the beeswax and anhydrous lanolin in a double boiler. Warm the pot marigold oil slightly in a second double boiler.

3 Combine the two mixtures and remove from the heat, stirring well.

4 When the mixture has started to cool significantly, but before it sets, add the tea tree oil. Stir. Pour into a sterilized, dark glass jar and allow the mixture to set.

APPLICATION *Rub gently on affected areas several times a day while symptoms persist.*

Boils & carbuncles

Boils occur when a hair follicle becomes inflamed and infected by bacteria. A cluster of boils is known as a carbuncle. Recurrent boils indicate weakened resistance to disease due to stress, exhaustion, or an underlying deep-seated infection, such as a dental abscess. Improving diet and lifestyle can help.

— SLIPPERY ELM POULTICE —

Hot poultices are very effective at drawing the core from boils. Slippery elm is ideal for this, with a few drops of eucalyptus oil added as an antiseptic.

~ INGREDIENTS ~
25 g powdered slippery elm (*Ulmus fulva*)
3 drops eucalyptus oil (*Eucalyptus globulus*)
water

~ HOW TO APPLY THE POULTICE ~

1 Add a little boiling water to the slippery elm powder to form a paste.

2 Mix in the eucalyptus oil.

3 Spread the hot mixture on the boil or carbuncle and cover with gauze. Reapply the hot mixture repeatedly each time the poultice cools, until the pus is discharged.

Supplementary treatments

■ To improve resistance to infection, take either 2 x 200 mg capsules of dried, powdered garlic or 5 ml of echinacea tincture (to make, see p. 68) 3 times a day.
■ Drink an infusion made from equal parts of dried honeysuckle flowers, figwort leaves, and thyme (to make, see p. 64) to help combat infection and cleanse the system.

Acne

Acne occurs most commonly in teenagers, and is characterized by blackheads, pustules, and cysts, caused by inflamed sebaceous glands in the skin. Poor diet is often a contributing factor. Although acne often clears by the time sufferers reach their early twenties, it can persist into middle age, possibly as a result of hormonal imbalance.

—— LAVENDER & YARROW FACIAL ——

In this two-part treatment, steam is used to open the pores and then a lotion is applied to cleanse the skin. The antiseptic and anti-inflammatory herbs that are added to the steam help to combat the symptoms of acne.

~ INGREDIENTS ~

5 drops tea tree oil (*Melaleuca alternifolia*)
25 ml rosewater (*Rosa damascena*)
25 ml distilled witch hazel (*Hamamelis virginiana*)
10 g dried lavender flowers (*Lavandula angustifolia*)
10 g dried yarrow flowers (*Achillea millefolium*)
10 g dried elderflowers (*Sambucus nigra*)
water

~ HOW TO MAKE THE FACIAL ~

1 Combine the tea tree oil with the rosewater and witch hazel to make an astringent lotion.

2 Mix the lavender, yarrow, and elderflowers in a basin and pour boiling water over them.

APPLICATION *Drape a towel over the head and basin and steam the face for 5–10 minutes, before cleansing with the lotion. Repeat once a day.*

Supplementary treatments

■ Take supplements of evening primrose oil, vitamin B-complex, vitamin C, and zinc (follow the instructions on the package), and eat plenty of fresh vegetables and fruit.
■ Blend 3 cabbage leaves with 50 ml distilled witch hazel in a food processor and use as a lotion twice a day.

Lavender

Yarrow

Dandruff

Small flakes of dead skin on the scalp, known as dandruff, can be a sign of psoriasis, although they are more commonly associated with seborrheic dermatitis or yeast infection.

—— ROSEMARY & NETTLE SHAMPOO ——

Rosemary is a stimulating, warming herb that is a traditional hair rinse, helping to keep hair shiny and healthy. Stinging nettle root is a favorite hair conditioner in many parts of Europe.

~ INGREDIENTS ~

25 g fresh rosemary leaves (*Rosmarinus officinalis*)
10 g fresh, well-washed, stinging nettle root (*Urtica dioica*)
5 drops tea tree oil (*Melaleuca alternifolia*)
20 g soft soap
100 ml denatured alcohol
350 ml water

~ HOW TO MAKE THE SHAMPOO ~

1 Mix the herbs, oil, soap, and alcohol in a 500 ml jar or wide-necked bottle. Add the water and shake well.

2 Leave to steep for 2 weeks, shaking at regular intervals. Strain into a clean bottle.

APPLICATION *Use as a shampoo 2 or 3 times a week until the dandruff disappears.*

Alopecia

As men age, gradual hair loss (baldness) often occurs. It tends to be hereditary and nonreversible. Where hair loss is sudden or patchy, as in alopecia, stress or vitamin deficiency may be to blame. It is found most commonly in teenagers and young adults.

Treatments

■ Apply arnica cream to the bald patches caused by alopecia (but do not use on broken skin).
■ Rinse the hair with standard infusions (to make, see p. 64) of rosemary, sage, or stinging nettle.
■ Take vitamin B and evening primrose oil supplements.
　■ If stress is a factor, drink an infusion of equal amounts of skullcap and wood betony (to make, see p. 64).

Cold sores

Once infected with the *Herpes simplex* virus, sufferers develop cold sores whenever the immune system is under stress. The sores usually occur in the same place, and are heralded by a prickling sensation in the skin. The best approach is to avoid recurrence by staying fit and healthy.

—— *TEA TREE & LAVENDER OIL* ——

Research has shown that a few herbs display specific antiviral properties and can be used topically to treat infections caused by viruses like Herpes simplex. *Use this lotion at the first suggestion of a cold sore.*

~ INGREDIENTS ~
8 ml tea tree oil (*Melaleuca alternifolia*)
5 ml lavender oil (*Lavandula angustifolia*)
12 ml sweet almond oil

~ HOW TO MAKE THE OIL ~

Combine the oils in a sterilized 25 ml dropper bottle and shake well.

APPLICATION *Dab 1–2 drops of the oil on the affected area. Repeat every 2 hours.*

Warts & verrucae

Caused by a viral infection, warts and verrucae can be very contagious. Many folk remedies exist – one of the simplest is to apply a few drops of fresh dandelion or greater celandine sap daily.

—— *THUJA & TEA TREE LOTION* ——

Thuja is a traditional remedy for treating warts and tea tree has powerful antiseptic and antifungal properties.

~ INGREDIENTS ~
15 ml thuja tincture (*Thuja occidentalis*)
10 ml tea tree oil (*Melaleuca alternifolia*)

~ HOW TO MAKE THE LOTION ~

To make the tincture, see p. 68. Combine the tincture and the oil in a sterilized 25 ml dropper bottle. Shake vigorously to form an emulsion.

APPLICATION *Dab 1–2 drops of the mix on the affected area. Repeat up to 4 times a day, shaking the bottle thoroughly before use.*

Impetigo

Impetigo is a common bacterial infection, usually affecting the mouth, nose, and ears, and producing a crusted discharge. It is highly contagious and is common in children. Topical use of antibiotics is often needed, but the following supplementary measures can help relieve the problem.

Treatments

■ Take 2 x 200 mg garlic capsules or 5 ml echinacea tincture (to make, see p. 68) 3 times a day.
■ Combine 20 ml echinacea tincture, 30 ml marigold tincture (to make, see p. 68), and 50 ml witch hazel, and use as a lotion, bathing the affected area 3 or 4 times a day.

Scabies

Scabies are tiny mites that burrow into the skin. They are highly contagious and irritating, and it is important to take professional advice. The following steps will help to combat the condition.

Treatments

■ Add 250 ml of a standard infusion of tansy (to make, see p. 64) to a hot bath at night. Combine 10 ml of tea tree oil and 90 ml of distilled witch hazel and use as a lotion after bathing. Repeat for 3 nights in a row.
■ Boil all clothing and bed linen and leave at least 3 weeks before using, as scabies' eggs can survive for 2 weeks.

CAUTION FOR IMPETIGO & SCABIES
• *Scabies and impetigo are extremely contagious: do not share towels or face cloths with the rest of the household.*

OVER-THE-COUNTER REMEDIES
Skin & Hair Problems

■ Many commercially available hair and skin beauty treatments contain herbal products. Usually the amount of herbal extract is far too small to be therapeutic, so look instead for more obviously medicinal products. Pot marigold cream is readily available, usually sold as calendula. Chickweed and chamomile creams and ointments are also produced commercially.
■ Cleansing herbs such as burdock, cleavers, dandelion, figwort, fumitory, and yellow dock are used in patent remedies for skin or hair problems. It is important to follow the instructions given, as most are digestive stimulants and excess intake can lead to diarrhea.
■ Soap bark is an excellent cleanser for dandruff.

ALLERGIES

IN OUR POLLUTED WORLD allergic reactions are all too common. The body has to cope with a growing variety of alien chemicals, due to ever-increasing levels of irritant exhaust fumes, as well as new strains of agricultural crops, such as rapeseed, and food that is often contaminated with pesticides and artificial growth stimulants. In response, the immune system treats the "unknowns" as dangerous, and inflammations and excessive mucus can result as part of the body's defense mechanisms.

Hay fever & allergic rhinitis

Usually triggered by seasonal grass or tree pollens, the familiar sneezing, sore eyes, and running nose characteristic of hay fever can also be caused by a reaction to house dust, car fumes, or animal hairs, when it is generally referred to as allergic rhinitis. Severe cases can lead to asthmalike symptoms.

— ELDERFLOWER & DANDELION TINCTURE —

Hay fever is often best treated in early spring, before the pollen arrives. This tincture, containing elderflower to strengthen the mucous membranes and dandelion to cleanse the liver, will help the system cope with future allergens and so reduce symptoms. This remedy is also suitable for allergic rhinitis.

~ INGREDIENTS ~

25 ml elderflower tincture (*Sambucus nigra*)
20 ml dandelion root tincture (*Taraxacum officinale*)
20 ml vervain tincture (*Verbena officinalis*)
15 ml Siberian ginseng tincture
(*Eleutherococcus senticosus*)
15 ml white horehound tincture (*Marrubium vulgare*)
5 ml licorice tincture (*Glycyrrhiza glabra*)

~ HOW TO MAKE THE TINCTURE ~

To make the individual tinctures, see p. 68. Mix the tinctures together in a 100 ml sterilized, dark glass bottle.

DOSAGE *Take 5 ml in 100 ml of warm water 3 times a day before meals. For hay fever, take for up to 4 weeks during the spring.*

Supplementary treatments

■ To relieve hay fever symptoms, bathe the eyes with Marigold & Eyebright Eyewash (see p. 93), and take 2 x 200 mg eyebright capsules up to 3 times a day.

Asthma

Allergic asthma is often linked with allergic eczema and starts in childhood. It is caused by a tightening of the small bronchial tubes and production of thick, sticky mucus that makes breathing difficult with a characteristic wheeze.

— SUNDEW & HYSSOP MIXTURE —

Use of many of the most effective herbs for asthma is restricted to professional practitioners and licensed, over-the-counter products. Sundew, an antispasmodic and relaxing expectorant, is one of the best generally available alternatives.

~ INGREDIENTS ~

10 ml sundew fluid extract (*Drosera rotundifolia*)
25 ml hyssop tincture (*Hyssopus officinalis*)
20 ml elecampane tincture (*Inula helenium*)
20 ml thyme tincture (*Thymus vulgaris*)
20 ml chamomile tincture (*Matricaria recutita*)
5 ml licorice fluid extract (*Glycyrrhiza glabra*)

~ HOW TO MAKE THE MIXTURE ~

To make the individual tinctures, see p. 68. Mix the ingredients in a 100 ml sterilized, dark glass bottle.

DOSAGE *Take 10 ml in 100 ml water twice a day before meals.*

CAUTION

• *This remedy should only be used for mild, stable conditions. Asthma can be life-threatening: seek professional help in severe cases. Do not suddenly stop using steroidal or other inhalants; their use should be phased out gradually only with professional help.*

Supplementary treatment

■ Use 5 drops of chamomile oil in a basin of boiling water as a steam inhalation (see p. 78) at the first hint of an attack.

Candidiasis

Candidiasis is the accelerated growth of yeastlike fungi, usually *Candida albicans*, which are naturally present in the gut. Candidiasis has been identified by some specialists as causing a wide variety of health problems, ranging from thrush and persistent urinary infections to panic attacks and chronic digestive disorders. Although some doctors remain sceptical, a low-sugar, yeast-free regime can help in many cases.

—— POT MARIGOLD & AGRIMONY TEA ——

Pot marigold is a good antifungal, both internally and externally, while agrimony helps to soothe the gut irritation caused by allergens and heal the mucous membranes.

~ INGREDIENTS ~

10 g dried echinacea root (*Echinacea angustifolia*)
600 ml water
10 g dried pot marigold petals (*Calendula officinalis*)
15 g dried agrimony leaves (*Agrimonia eupatoria*)

~ HOW TO MAKE THE TEA ~

1 Simmer the echinacea root in the water for 10 minutes to make a decoction.

2 Mix the pot marigold and agrimony in a teapot and pour on the freshly made decoction. Steep for 10 minutes. Strain into a jug and cover. The surplus may be kept in a cool place or refrigerator for up to 48 hours.

DOSAGE *Drink a wineglass dose 3 times a day before meals until the infection clears. Do not sweeten the tea with honey or sugar while on a yeast-free diet – try a squeeze of fresh lemon juice or 1–2 drops of peppermint essence instead.*

Supplementary treatments

■ Garlic is an antifungal herb. Take 1–2 x 200 mg capsules 3 times a day or use plenty of garlic in cooking.
■ Take 1 g of evening primrose oil in capsules and 1–2 capsules containing lactobacillus bacteria (e.g., *L. bifidus* and *L. acidophilus*) daily.
■ Avoid yeast extracts, fungi-based foods (e.g. mycoproteins, mushrooms), sugars, dairy products, alcohol, refined carbohydrates, junk food, and preserved foods. Avoid excessive amounts of fruit.
■ Candidiasis can give rise to a wide range of symptoms. Select infusions and additional treatments to match the pattern of symptoms. See pp. 116–17 for joint pain and pp. 102–7 for digestive remedies.

Food intolerance

Food sensitivity often starts in childhood with the introduction of cow's milk, which is a protein alien to the developing digestive system. If possible, breastfeed babies for the first 4 months, or use soy-based formulas. Food intolerance can cause chronic digestive disturbances, arthritislike symptoms, eczema, asthma, and ear problems. Eliminating the problem food is essential; in the meantime, herbs help repair the system and increase tolerance.

—— MARSHMALLOW & LEMON BALM TEA ——

Soothing marshmallow coats and protects the gut, and lemon balm is a carminative, ideal for digestive upsets.

~ INGREDIENTS ~

5 g dried marshmallow root (*Althaea officinalis*)
5 g fenugreek seeds (*Trigonella foenum-graecum*)
10 g dried *Dang Shen* (*Codonopsis pilosula*)
750 ml water
10 g dried or 30 g fresh lemon balm leaves
(*Melissa officinalis*)
10 g dried agrimony (*Agrimonia eupatoria*)

~ HOW TO MAKE THE TEA ~

1 Simmer the marshmallow, fenugreek, and *Dang Shen* in water for 15–20 minutes to make a decoction.

2 Put the lemon balm and agrimony in a teapot and pour on the freshly made decoction. Steep for 10 minutes. Strain into a jug and cover.

DOSAGE *Drink a wineglass dose 4 times a day.*

Supplementary treatments

■ It is essential to identify the problem food. Seek professional help or try to eliminate these possible allergens for 2 weeks: milk and milk products, wheat, red meat, salicylates, tomatoes, potatoes, and peppers.

OVER-THE-COUNTER REMEDIES
Allergies

■ Look for patent hay fever remedies that contain eyebright, or goldenseal.
■ Various remedies for candidiasis are available, although so far there is little evidence to support their claims. They may contain biotin, caprylic acid and derivatives, echinacea extracts, evening primrose oil, linseed oil, and tea tree oil.

DIGESTIVE PROBLEMS

WE ARE NOT ONLY WHAT WE EAT, but also what we digest. Keeping the digestive system in good working order is a vital part of staying healthy, since failure to extract the necessary nutrients from food, or to excrete surplus wastes, can lead to all sorts of health problems, such as vitamin or mineral deficiencies, arthritic or skin problems associated with toxins lingering in the system, or headaches.

Fresh hop aerial parts

Dried wild yam root

Irritable bowel syndrome

Irritable bowel syndrome is a common label for a wide range of gastric symptoms, generally characterized by alternating diarrhea and constipation, as well as gas, abdominal bloating, and pain. It is commonly related to stress or food intolerance (see p. 101).

WILD YAM ROOT *is a muscle relaxant that eases the colicky pains associated with irritable bowel syndrome.*

Wild yam root tincture

—— WILD YAM & CHAMOMILE MIXTURE ——

Wild yam is an effective antispasmodic that helps to relax the gut and relieve the overactivity contributing to the problem. Hops and chamomile act as relaxants, while the bitterness of hops helps restore normal digestion.

~ INGREDIENTS ~
30 ml wild yam root tincture (*Dioscorea villosa*)
30 ml chamomile flower tincture (*Matricaria recutita*)
20 ml bistort tincture (*Polygonum bistorta*)
15 ml hop tincture (*Humulus lupulus*)
5 ml licorice fluid extract (*Glycyrrhiza glabra*)

~ HOW TO MAKE THE MIXTURE ~
To make the individual tinctures, see p. 68. Pour the tinctures and fluid extract into a 100 ml sterilized, dark glass bottle and shake.

DOSAGE *Take 5 ml in 100 ml of warm water 3 times a day until symptoms ease.*

Chamomile flower tincture

Fresh chamomile flowers

CHAMOMILE FLOWERS *help to counteract stress, which is often a factor in irritable bowel syndrome. They calm the nerves and the digestive system.*

Fresh bistort aerial parts

Dried bistort root

Bistort tincture

BISTORT *was once known as "snakeroot." It is a helpful astringent for soothing gut inflammation.*

HOPS *are a bitter stimulant and a sedative, helping to regulate digestion and calm the nerves.*

Fresh hops

Hop tincture

Chopped dried licorice root

Dried licorice root

LICORICE *reduces inflammation and helps to stimulate and restore the digestion.*

Licorice fluid extract

SUPPLEMENTARY TREATMENTS

■ Chamomile infusion (to make, see p. 64) taken regularly can aid relaxation and calm gut spasms.
■ Cramp bark tincture is a potent antispasmodic (to make, see p. 68). Take 5–10 drops at 30–60 minute intervals to help relieve abdominal cramps. Meadowsweet tincture can also help. Take up to 5 ml diluted in 100 ml of warm water 3 times a day.
■ If the condition appears to be linked to the menstrual cycle, evening primrose oil may be of benefit. Take 2 x 500 mg capsules a day

CAUTIONS FOR DIGESTIVE PROBLEMS

- *Seek professional help for any persistent or severe abdominal pains, or if bowel patterns change significantly.*
- *Avoid excessive or prolonged use of licorice if suffering from high blood pressure (seek professional advice).*
- *Do not use strong laxatives in pregnancy.*

WILD YAM & CHAMOMILE MIXTURE is a calming remedy, which eases stress, relaxes abdominal cramps, and restores the digestive tract to health.

Wild yam & chamomile mixture

Constipation

Failure to empty the bowels regularly can be linked to a lack of dietary fiber or to a sluggish digestion. In the West, it can take 72 hours for food to pass through us, as against an average of 12 in developing countries, where food is less highly processed.

— LICORICE & DANDELION DECOCTION —

Chronic constipation often suggests a sluggish digestion, which can be improved by bitter herbs that stimulate the liver and encourage production of digestive enzymes. Dandelion is a good liver tonic, while yellow dock has a gentle laxative action.

~ INGREDIENTS ~

10 g dried dandelion root (*Taraxacum officinale*)
5 g dried yellow dock root (*Rumex crispus*)
5 g dried licorice root (*Glycyrrhiza glabra*)
5 g dried anise seeds (*Pimpinella anisum*)
750 ml water

~ HOW TO MAKE THE DECOCTION ~

1 Put the herbs in a pan and add the water.

2 Bring to a boil and simmer gently for 10 minutes, or until the volume has reduced by approximately one-third. Strain into a jug. Cover, and store in a cool place.

DOSAGE *Take a wineglass dose 3 times a day.*

CAUTIONS
• *Recurrent constipation can indicate more serious underlying health conditions. Seek professional advice before resorting to persistent or excessive use of laxatives.*
• *Do not use strong laxatives, e.g., senna or rhubarb, in pregnancy.*

Supplementary treatments
■ Get regular exercise and drink plenty of fluids, including a glass of warm water first thing in the morning.
■ Psyllium husks and seeds can help to lubricate the bowel, easing the passage of dry, hard stools. Add a teaspoon of seeds to a cup of boiling water. Steep for 10 minutes, stir well, and drink the entire mix first thing in the morning.
■ Rhubarb root is a potent laxative. Take 10–20 drops of the tincture (to make, see p. 68) in 100 ml of warm water 3 times a day before meals for chronic problems. If pregnant, use butternut in the same way.
■ If tension is part of the problem, take 2–3 ml of cramp bark tincture in 100 ml of warm water before meals.

Fennel

Chamomile   *Fennel & chamomile tea*

Flatulence

Gas – traveling in either direction – can be a symptom of various digestive ailments, such as gastritis, gallbladder problems, or irritable bowel syndrome (see p. 102). It can also be associated with poor diet, nervousness, or stress. Carminative herbs after meals can help, but professional advice may be needed to identify the cause of the problem.

——— FENNEL & CHAMOMILE TEA ———

The calming and anti-inflammatory actions of fennel and chamomile provide a soothing mixture for the relief of gas. This is also a palatable after-dinner infusion, suitable for regular use.

~ INGREDIENTS ~

25 g dried fennel seeds (*Foeniculum officinalis*)
25 g dried chamomile flowers (*Matricaria recutita*)
10 g dried peppermint aerial parts (*Mentha piperita*)
water

~ HOW TO MAKE THE TEA ~

1 Mix the herbs and store in a dry, airtight container.

2 Put 2-3 teaspoons of the mix in a tisane cup or small teapot. Add a cup of freshly boiled water and steep for 5-10 minutes. Strain.

DOSAGE *Drink a cup regularly after meals.*

Supplementary treatments
■ Many culinary herbs aid digestion: add anise, dill, fennel, or lemon balm to dishes, and cook with warm spices such as ginger, fenugreek, caraway, or cayenne.
■ If symptoms are severe, massage the abdomen with a mixture of 2 drops of cinnamon or clove oil in 10 ml of sweet almond oil.

Diarrhea

Diarrhea, characterized by loose and frequent stools, is generally a symptom of imbalance rather than a primary disease. Food poisoning or bacterial infections are often responsible for sudden attacks, and the aim of treatment is to help the body to rid itself of toxins, rather than simply suppressing the symptoms.

Tormentil & Marshmallow Decoction

This mixture of herbs and arrowroot is soothing and nutritious. Tormentil root is rich in tannins and highly astringent, helping to reduce inflammation, while marshmallow is soothing.

~ Ingredients ~

1 tablespoon arrowroot
15 g dried tormentil root (*Potentilla erecta*)
10 g dried marshmallow root (*Althaea officinalis*)
5 g dried cinnamon bark (*Cinnamomum zeylanicum*)
750 ml water

~ How to make the decoction ~

1 Blend the arrowroot with a tablespoon of cold water to form a paste in a bowl or jug.

2 Simmer the herbs in the water for 10–15 minutes. Strain, return the liquid to the pan, and bring to a boil.

3 Pour the boiling decoction over the blended arrowroot stirring well. Store the surplus in a cool place.

Dosage *Take a teacup dose 3 times a day until symptoms subside. Sweeten with honey if required.*

Bistort & Agrimony Tincture

Diarrhea can be a problem on vacation, with strange foods and unfamiliar bugs. This mixture is useful to pack in the luggage for emergencies. Both agrimony and bistort are astringent herbs, helpful for treating diarrhea.

~ Ingredients ~

25 ml bistort tincture (*Polygonum bistorta*)
35 ml agrimony tincture (*Agrimonia eupatoria*)
20 ml marshmallow tincture (*Althaea officinalis*)
10 ml *Lian Qiao* tincture (forsythia berries – *Forsythia suspensa*)
10 ml *Jin Yin Hua* (*Lonicera japonica*)

~ How to make the tincture ~

Make the individual tinctures, see p. 68. Mix the tinctures in a sterilized, dark glass bottle.

Dosage *Take 10 ml of the tincture in 100 ml of warm water 3 times a day when symptoms are acute. Repeat for up to 3 days.*

Caution

• *Seek professional help if diarrhea persists for more than 2 or 3 days (or more than 24 hours in babies or toddlers); if it is accompanied by fever; or if there is blood or mucus in the stool.*

Fresh marshmallow

Dried marshmallow root

Dried tormentil root

Supplementary treatments

■ Drink cups of strong, cool, black Indian tea, without milk or sugar, to reduce inflammation in the gut.
■ Meadowsweet tincture (to make, see p. 68) can be very soothing for gut inflammation. Take 2 ml in warm water at hourly intervals up to 10 times a day.
■ An infusion (to make, see p. 64) of agrimony can be helpful. Drink a cup 3 or 4 times a day.

Hemorrhoids

Hemorrhoids, or piles, are varicose veins in the wall of the rectum, frequently associated with a poor diet, constipation, or liver imbalance. They also may occur during pregnancy. They often bleed and may be inflamed. Increasing dietary intake of fruit and vegetables can help.

─── PILEWORT OINTMENT ───

In the Middle Ages the nodular roots of the lesser celandine plant reminded people of the appearance of piles – hence the traditional, alternative name for the herb. Pilewort is a very astringent plant, and can be extremely helpful for hemorrhoids.

~ INGREDIENTS ~
75 g dried pilewort leaves (*Ranunculus ficaria*)
500 ml sunflower oil
25 g beeswax
25 g anhydrous lanolin

~ HOW TO MAKE THE OINTMENT ~

1 Heat the pilewort and the oil in a double boiler, or over a waterbath, for 3 hours to make an infused oil, and strain the mixture through a jelly bag (see p. 73).

2 Meanwhile, melt the beeswax and anhydrous lanolin in a separate saucepan.

3 Add 100 ml of the warm infused oil to the melted mixture in the saucepan. Stir well and pour the ointment into sterilized jars before it starts to set.

APPLICATION *Gently rub the ointment on affected areas several times a day.*

Supplementary treatments
■ If the piles are irritated or bleeding, apply a little distilled witch hazel on a cotton pad to the affected area.
■ Drink an infusion (see p. 64) made from equal amounts of yarrow, linden flowers, and melilot to help improve venous circulation.
■ Avoid constipation, which exacerbates hemorrhoids – follow the recommendations on p. 104.

Gastritis

Gastritis, or inflammation of the stomach lining, is a common result of "overindulgence" or upsetting foods, and can lead to nausea, vomiting, diarrhea, and heartburn. Symptoms are usually short-lived.

─── MEADOWSWEET TEA ───

Meadowsweet is a cooling and very soothing herb, which eases inflammation and helps to reduce acidic secretions in the stomach.

~ INGREDIENTS ~
25 g meadowsweet (*Filipendula ulmaria*)
500 ml water

~ HOW TO MAKE THE TEA ~

Place the herb in a teapot. Add freshly boiled water and leave to steep for 10 minutes. Strain the surplus into a covered jug and store in a cool place.

DOSAGE *Sip a large mugful of the mixture when symptoms are acute. Flavor with a little honey or licorice juice if required. Repeat if necessary.*

CAUTION
• *Avoid excessive use of meadowsweet in cases of aspirin allergy.*

Supplementary treatments
■ Meadowsweet tincture (to make, see p. 68) can be used as an alternative to the tea. Take 2 ml in warm water every hour while symptoms persist, up to 10 times a day.
■ Take 2–3 slippery elm capsules every couple of hours while symptoms are severe.
■ If the gastritis is linked to a hangover, take 5 ml of milk thistle tincture and 2 x 500 mg capsules of evening primrose oil. Repeat every 3 hours while symptoms continue, for up to 12 hours.

Meadowsweet

Fennel & lemon balm tea

Fennel   *Lemon balm*

Indigestion & heartburn

Eating too quickly, or while sitting awkwardly, can often lead to indigestion. If it is a regular problem, then some underlying digestive imbalance may be to blame. Heartburn is a common problem in pregnancy and obesity, and it can also be a side-effect of some orthodox medication.

FENNEL & LEMON BALM TEA

Both these herbs are very calming for the stomach, while lemon balm also helps relax the nerves if stress or anxiety is contributing to the problem.

~ INGREDIENTS ~
10 g dried fennel seeds (*Foeniculum officinalis*)
15 g dried, or 45 g fresh lemon balm leaves
(*Melissa officinalis*)
2–3 g dried cinnamon bark or a pinch of powdered
cinnamon (*Cinnamomum zeylanicum*)
500 ml water

~ HOW TO MAKE THE TEA ~
Place the herbs in a teapot. Add freshly boiled water and leave to steep for 10 minutes. Strain into a covered jug. The surplus may be stored in a cool place for up to 48 hours.

DOSAGE *Take in wineglass doses after meals as required.*

Supplementary treatments
■ Slippery elm capsules or 5 g of the powdered bark stirred into a cup of water can soothe heartburn.
■ Take carminative teas regularly. Try chamomile, peppermint, fennel, or lemon balm (to make, see p. 64).

Nausea & vomiting

Nausea and vomiting are common symptoms of digestive upsets, fevers, and migraines. Many people also suffer from nausea in early pregnancy, or when traveling.

GINGER CAPSULES

Ginger in almost any form is excellent for nausea and vomiting. Crystallized ginger, ginger beer, ginger wine, or even ginger cookies, can all be useful if nothing else is available. The herb has been shown to be safe and effective, even in pregnancy.

~ INGREDIENTS ~
50 g powdered ginger (*Zingiber officinalis*)
size 00 gelatin or vegetarian capsules

~ HOW TO MAKE THE CAPSULES ~
1 Pour the powdered ginger into a saucer.

2 Separate the 2 halves of a capsule case and slide them together through the powder, scooping it into the capsule. Join the 2 halves together.

DOSAGE *Take 2 capsules every couple of hours while symptoms persist.*

Supplementary treatments
■ Tinctures of black horehound, chamomile, cloves, ginger, or greater celandine can help nausea. Keeping remedies down can be a problem in cases of severe nausea and vomiting. Try placing a couple of drops of tincture on the tongue for rapid absorption.

OVER-THE-COUNTER REMEDIES
Digestive Problems

■ Senna leaves and pods are readily available in tablets and capsules for constipation. This herb should be taken on an occasional basis, since it works by irritating the digestive tract to encourage movement. Excessive use can weaken the gut with long-term use. Avoid during pregnancy.
■ Slippery elm capsules are helpful for gastritis and indigestion. They are readily available from health food stores.
■ Many "after-dinner" herbal tea blends contain digestive stimulants that can help regulate activity. Herbs used commercially include: barberry, boldo leaves (a liver stimulant), dandelion, and vervain.

CIRCULATORY DISORDERS

HEART DISEASE and other circulatory problems are widespread in the developed world, due in part to sedentary lifestyles, diets that are over-rich in saturated animal fats, smoking, and excessive stress. Regular exercise and a healthy diet can help, as can simple herbal remedies, such as garlic and oat bran to reduce cholesterol levels and linden to ease stress and combat artherosclerosis.

Poor circulation

Poor circulation can be an inherited condition, although it is also common among the elderly and those who have become run-down and exhausted. Cold weather may make things worse, because as small arteries constrict, blood flow is restricted, leading to blue fingers and toes.

——— GINGER & CINNAMON TEA ———

Herbs that stimulate the circulation, such as cinnamon and ginger, are generally hot and spicy. The Chinese regard Gui Zhi *(cinnamon twigs) as the most effective part of the herb for sending heat to the peripheries, but the more familiar cinnamon stick (made from the bark) can be substituted if twigs are unavailable.*

~ INGREDIENTS ~

15 g fresh ginger root, sliced (*Zingiber officinalis*)
10 g *Gui Zhi* (cinnamon twigs – *Cinnamomum cassia*)
10 g dried angelica root (*Angelica archangelica*)
700 ml water

~ HOW TO MAKE THE TEA ~

Heat the herbs and the water in a pan and simmer for 10–15 minutes. Strain into a covered jug. The surplus can be stored in a cool place for up to 48 hours.

DOSAGE *Drink a teacup dose while it is hot. Take a dose 3 times a day, reheating the tea each time.*

Supplementary treatments

■ Use arnica cream (to make, see p. 76) or drops of arnica tincture (to make, see p. 68) on unbroken skin.
■ Drink buckwheat infusion regularly (to make see p. 64) or take rutin tablets to help strengthen the circulation.
■ Foot or hand baths can be helpful. Soak the affected part in hot water and 10 ml of mustard powder.

High blood pressure

Raised blood pressure needs professional investigation since it may be a sign of heart, liver, or kidney disease. Many cases have no obvious cause, and herbs can provide a valuable alternative to orthodox remedies.

— HAWTHORN & CHRYSANTHEMUM TEA —

Hawthorn helps to improve the coronary circulation, making the heart more efficient, while chrysanthemum flowers relax the heart and improve blood flow. This mixture is ideal for mild conditions.

~ INGREDIENTS ~

30 g dried hawthorn flowering tops (*Crataegus oxyacantha*)
25 g *Ju Hua* (dried, prepared chrysanthemum flowers – *Chrysanthemum morifolium*)
25 g dried linden flowers (*Tilia europaea*)
20 g dried yarrow (*Achillea millefolium*)
water

~ HOW TO MAKE THE TEA ~

1 Mix the herbs and store in a dry, airtight container.

2 Place 2 teaspoons of the mix in a tisane cup or small teapot. Add a cup of freshly boiled water and steep for 10 minutes. Strain.

DOSAGE *Drink a teacup dose 3 times a day.*

CAUTIONS

• *Omit the yarrow if pregnant. Maintain regular blood pressure checks, and do not replace long-term orthodox medication with herbs before first consulting a doctor or herbal practitioner.*

Supplementary treatment

■ Eliminate tea, coffee, and alcohol from the diet and avoid added salt. Take 400 IU vitamin E daily.

Varicose veins

Progress of the blood through the veins on its return to the heart depends largely on muscle contractions. Lack of exercise, pregnancy, or obesity can make the return tortuous: vessel walls weaken and blood stagnates leading to varicose veins, which can be seen as twisted, swollen veins on the skin's surface.

—— STINGING NETTLE & MELILOT TEA ——

Herbs rich in silica, such as stinging nettle and horsetail, help strengthen the vein walls, as do herbs such as shepherd's purse and buckwheat, which contain bioflavonoids.

~ INGREDIENTS ~
10 g dried stinging nettle (*Urtica dioica*)
10 g dried melilot (*Melilotus officinalis*)
10 g dried shepherd's purse (*Capsella bursa-pastoris*)
or buckwheat (*Fagopyrum esculentum*)
20 ml horsetail juice (*Equisetum arvense*)
500 ml water

~ HOW TO MAKE THE TEA ~

1 Use commercially prepared horsetail juice, or make a decoction by simmering 60 g of fresh herb in 750 ml water for at least 3 hours, adding water as necessary.

2 Mix the dried herbs together in a teapot or lidded jug and add the freshly boiled water. Steep for 15 minutes and strain.

3 Add the horsetail juice or 100 ml of the homemade decoction to the infusion and stir well.

DOSAGE *Take a wineglass dose 3 times a day before meals.*

Supplementary treatments
■ Raise the foot of the bed by 10–15 cm.
■ Use compresses (see p. 71) of chilled, distilled witch hazel or horsechestnut tincture (to make, see p. 68) to ease the discomfort of varicose veins.

Stinging nettle   *Melilot*

Iron-deficient anemia

Iron is needed to make hemoglobin, which transports oxygen around the body in the blood. Its lack leads to anemia characterized by fatigue, breathlessness, pallor, dizziness, and rheumatic-like pains. Anemia is common, especially among women with heavy periods.

—— APRICOT IRON TONIC ——

Apricots are rich in iron and are a good base for this tonic. Stinging nettles and dandelion are added to provide extra nutrients and to stimulate the liver.

~ INGREDIENTS ~
250 g fresh apricots
(organically grown if possible)
500 ml water
1 liter red wine
250 g honey or sugar
100 ml stinging nettle tincture or juice (*Urtica dioica*)
50 ml dandelion root tincture (*Taraxacum officinale*)

~ HOW TO MAKE THE TONIC ~

1 To make the tinctures, see p. 68.

2 Put the apricots and water in a pan and bring to a boil. Transfer to a slow cooker and simmer for 12 hours.

3 Allow to cool and remove the stones. Blend in a food processor to produce a fruit pulp.

4 Add the red wine and herb tinctures and stir well. Store in sterilized, dark glass bottles for up to 3 months.

DOSAGE *Take 10 ml twice a day.*

CAUTION
● *Alcoholic mixtures should be avoided during pregnancy. Drink a daily cup of stinging nettle tea instead (to make, see p. 64).*

OVER-THE-COUNTER REMEDIES
Circulatory Disorders

■ For anemia, try preparations rich in *Dang Gui* – often sold as a woman's tonic herb – to help nourish the blood. (*Dang Gui* should be avoided in pregnancy.)
■ *Ginkgo biloba* features as a circulatory herb in many over-the-counter mixtures. It is most useful as a remedy for cerebral circulation, but is also helpful for atherosclerosis, which contributes to raised blood pressure.
■ Rutin tablets help strengthen the circulation.

HEADACHES, MIGRAINES & NEURALGIA

HEADACHES ARE GENERALLY a sign that the body is out of balance. Those that seem to be focused behind the eyes are often characteristic of digestive problems. If they are in the front of the face, along the cheekbones, they may be part of a sinus disorder. Headaches that seem to start at the back of the neck and gradually creep over the skull are often tension related. It is essential to treat the cause, which can mean changing eating habits or learning to relax.

GENERAL CAUTION
• *Seek professional advice if headaches are recurrent or sustained, as they can be a symptom of high blood pressure and other conditions.*

Tension headaches

Tension headaches start at the end of a long day or when stress begins to mount. If possible, take a break from the task in hand – go for a short walk, or spend a few minutes brewing a relaxing and soothing tea, and then take time to drink it slowly.

—— *WOOD BETONY TEA* ——

This relaxing mixture is based on wood betony, one of the most popular medicinal herbs in medieval times. The herb is a potent painkiller and relaxant.

~ INGREDIENTS ~
30 g dried wood betony (*Stachys betonia*)
10 g dried chamomile (*Matricaria recutita*)
10 g dried skullcap (*Scutellaria lateriflora*)
water

~ HOW TO MAKE THE TEA ~
1 Mix the herbs and store in a dry, airtight container.

2 Place 2 teaspoons of the mixed herbs in a tisane cup or small teapot. Add freshly boiled water and steep for 5–10 minutes. Strain.

DOSAGE *Drink a teacup dose every hour until the headache subsides.*

Supplementary treatment
■ Add 2 drops of lavender oil to a warm bath and relax.
■ Take 2–3 drops of wood betony or lavender tincture (to make, see p. 68) on the tongue at first sign of the headache. Repeat every 20–30 minutes while symptoms persist.

Sinus headaches

Thick phlegm blocking the sinus cavities in the skull around the nose, eyes, and cheeks can lead to severe head pain, which is persistent in some cases. The pain can extend to the upper jaw, simulating toothache.

—— *LAVENDER & PINE INHALATION* ——

Steam inhalations are a good way to clear mucus. This mixture contains potent essential oils, which reduce inflammation and infection.

~ INGREDIENTS ~
water
10 drops lavender oil (*Lavandula angustifolia*)
5 drops pine oil (*Pinus sylvestris*)
5 drops eucalyptus oil (*Eucalyptus globulus*)
5 drops thyme oil (*Thymus vulgaris*)

~ HOW TO USE THE INHALATION ~
1 Fill a large basin or mixing bowl with boiling water. Add the essential oils.

2 Lean over the water and cover the head and basin with a towel. Inhale the steam for 10 minutes. Repeat 2 or 3 times a day.
Note: Stay in a warm room for 30 minutes after each inhalation.

Supplementary treatments
■ If the sinus areas are not too painful, gently massage elderflower cream (to make, see p. 76) across the nose and cheeks 2 or 3 times a day. See also p. 90 for advice on treating sinusitis.

Migraines

Migraines are severe headaches, often characterized by eye disturbances, such as flashing lights at the edge of the field of vision, as well as pins and needles in the arms and hands, and possibly nausea and vomiting. Stress, food intolerance, and menstrual irregularities can all be trigger factors, and it is important to identify and treat the cause.

—— *FEVERFEW & VALERIAN TINCTURE* ——

Modern research has shown feverfew to be effective for treating migraine. Eating fresh leaves can prevent attacks, although the taste of the plant is extremely bitter.

~ INGREDIENTS ~

10 ml feverfew tincture (*Tanacetum parthenium*)
10 ml valerian tincture (*Valeriana officinalis*)
5 ml lavender tincture (*Lavandula angustifolia*)

~ HOW TO MAKE THE TINCTURE ~

To make the individual tinctures, see p. 68. Combine them in a sterilized dropper bottle.

DOSAGE *Drink 15–20 drops of the tincture in a little warm water. Repeat at 15–60 minute intervals while symptoms persist.*

CAUTIONS

- *Do not use feverfew if taking warfarin or other blood-thinning drugs.*
- *Feverfew can cause mouth ulcers. Do not use if this happens.*

Supplementary treatments

■ At the first signs of a migraine, massage a little of a mixture made from 20 drops lavender oil and 10 ml sweet almond oil into the nape of the neck and the temples.
■ See if a cold compress applied to the head eases the migraine (to make, see p. 71). If so, drinking lavender infusion can also help (to make, see p. 64). Other types of migraine respond to a hot towel on the forehead, in which case drink rosemary infusion (to make, see p. 64).

Dried lavender

Neuralgia

Inflammation of the facial nerves is often caused by chills and drafts, and occurs most commonly when the sufferer is tired and run down. The pain from the affected nerve, known as neuralgia, is severe and localized along the path of the nerve. The skin is usually extremely sensitive to touch.

—— *ST.-JOHN'S-WORT & LAVENDER TEA* ——

St.-John's-wort is a good restorative for the nervous system, helping to reduce inflammation, and lavender is a soothing herb that is frequently used to treat nervous complaints.

~ INGREDIENTS ~

15 g dried St.-John's-wort (*Hypericum perfoliatum*)
10 g dried lavender flowers (*Lavandula angustifolia*)
500 ml water

~ HOW TO MAKE THE TEA ~

1. Mix the herbs together in a teapot.

2. Pour on the freshly boiled water and steep for 10 minutes. Strain into a jug with a lid and store the surplus in a cool place for up to 48 hours.

DOSAGE *Slowly sip a large mug of the hot tea. Reheat the tea and continue sipping it while the symptoms are severe.*

CAUTION

- *Seek professional help immediately if the area is very inflamed or hot, suggesting an acute infection, or if there is any paralysis or stiffness associated with the pain.*

Supplementary treatments

■ Very gently pat a little of a mixture made from 5 drops lemon oil and 10 ml sweet almond oil on to the skin.
■ A hot compress soaked in an infusion made from St.-John's-wort and vervain may help (to make, see p. 71).

OVER-THE-COUNTER REMEDIES
Headaches, Migraines & Neuralgia

■ For tension headaches, look for combinations of these relaxing herbs in capsules or tablets: California poppy, chamomile, Jamaican dogwood, lemon balm, linden flowers, skullcap, and valerian.
■ Feverfew capsules for migraines are readily available.
■ Elderflower teabags are available commercially and can be a convenient aid for sinus headaches.

MIND & EMOTIONS

STRESS IS A NORMAL part of life; the human body is designed to cope with regular rises in tension levels as the "flight or fight" hormone, epinephrine, prepares us for action. Problems arise when these peaks are sustained for too long. A perpetual state of alertness brings exhaustion and an inability to relax and unwind. It is important to tackle the underlying causes, since prolonged stress can cause emotional upsets and problems, such as depression and anxiety. If left untreated, stress can start to affect bodily functions, often leading to digestive disorders, headaches, or lack of libido.

Coping with stress

Stress is blamed for a multitude of ills, but researchers believe that everyone needs a certain amount to function properly. Too much stress can be damaging, so it is important to learn when to take a break. Brewing a soothing herbal tea and taking time to sip it slowly is a good way to help the body unwind.

—— WOOD BETONY & LINDEN TEA ——

Wood betony was traditionally prescribed for the fearful and is a good restorative. Linden flowers, often used for heart-related disorders, are a nervine and can help prevent stress-related problems.

~ INGREDIENTS ~

20 g dried wood betony (*Stachys betonica*)
10 g dried linden flowers (*Tilia europaea*)
10 g dried chamomile flowers (*Matricaria recutita*)
10 g dried *gotu kola* (*Centella asiatica*)
water

~ HOW TO MAKE THE TEA ~

1 Mix the herbs and store in a dry, airtight container.

2 Put 2 teaspoons in a tisane cup or small teapot and add freshly boiled water. Steep for 5–10 minutes. Strain.

DOSAGE *Drink a teacup dose 3 or 4 times a day as required.*

Supplementary treatments
■ Take 2–3 x 200 mg tablets of Siberian ginseng a day several weeks before likely stressful periods, and continue until stress levels revert to normal.
■ Add 5 drops of lavender, basil, or sandalwood oil to the bathwater at night. (Do not use basil oil in pregnancy.)

Anxiety & tension

Irritability, tears, headaches, and sleeplessness can all be signs of anxiety and tension. Identifying the cause of the problem is vital, as is learning to relax and unwind. Take 10 minutes a day to practice deep breathing exercises, use visualization tapes, or find time to meditate somewhere peaceful.

— SKULLCAP & PASSIONFLOWER MIXTURE —

Soothing herbal nervines encourage relaxation and reduce tensions. Skullcap is a restorative and relaxant, while passionflower has an effective sedative action.

~ INGREDIENTS ~

50 ml skullcap tincture (*Scutellaria lateriflora*)
25 ml passionflower tincture (*Passiflora incarnata*)
15 ml lemon balm tincture (*Melissa officinalis*)
10 ml pasque flower tincture (*Anemone vulgaris*)

~ HOW TO MAKE THE MIXTURE ~

To make the individual tinctures, see p. 68. Mix the tinctures together in a 100 ml sterilized, dark glass bottle.

DOSAGE *Take 5 ml in a little warm water when feeling anxious and tense. Repeat up to 5 times a day.*

Supplementary treatments
■ If symptoms include panic attacks, try massaging 5 drops of rose or neroli oil diluted in a teaspoon of sweet almond oil into the temples.
■ Bach Flower Remedies can be helpful for emotional tensions. Try red chestnut for worries about other people, elm for doubt in abilities, and vervain for stress. Put 4 drops in a 10 ml dropper bottle of water and take 1–2 drops on the tongue at frequent intervals.

Depression

Everyone experiences emotional ups and downs, but when the downs turn into severe depression expert help is often needed to lift the spirits. Associated symptoms can include constipation, lack of concentration, and a desire to withdraw from human company and say little.

——— LEMON BALM & OAT MIXTURE ———

Oats are a good antidepressant and restorative for the nervous system and combine well with vervain. Lemon balm is a relaxant for the central nervous system. St.-John's-wort is another effective nervous system remedy, widely used in Europe as an antidepressant.

~ INGREDIENTS ~

30 ml oat tincture (*Avena sativa*)
25 ml St.-John's-wort tincture (*Hypericum perforatum*)
25 ml vervain tincture (*Verbena officinalis*)
15 ml lemon balm tincture (*Melissa officinalis*)
5 ml licorice tincture (*Glycyrrhiza glabra*)

~ HOW TO MAKE THE MIXTURE ~

To make the individual tinctures, see p. 68. Mix the tinctures together in a 100 ml sterilized, dark glass bottle.

DOSAGE *Take 5–10 ml in a little warm water 3 times a day before meals.*

Supplementary treatments

■ Drink an infusion of wood betony and basil. Mix together equal amounts of dried basil and wood betony and store in a dry, airtight container. Make an infusion (see p. 64) using 1–2 teaspoons of the mix to a cup of water.
■ Use gorse, mustard, or gentian Bach Flower Remedies. Put 4 drops of the flower remedy in a 10 ml dropper bottle of water and take 1–2 drops on the tongue at frequently.
■ Add 5 drops of basil or sandalwood oil to the bathwater. (Do not use basil oil in pregnancy.)

Insomnia

Overexcitement, worries, illness – the causes of sleeplessness are many and identifying contributing factors is vital. The pattern of insomnia is also important: is the problem an over-active mind preventing sleep? Is restless, light sleep causing wakefulness in the early hours? In both cases relaxing in a warm bath before bed can often help.

——— NIGHTCAP & PASSIONFLOWER TEA ———

California poppies are sometimes known as "nightcap" and were once used as a sedative remedy by Native Americans. Like other poppies, they contain potent alkaloids, but these are far less powerful than the morphine of opium poppy, giving a gentle soothing remedy that is safe to use, even for children.

~ INGREDIENTS ~

20 g dried California poppy (*Eschscholzia californica*)
15 g dried passionflower (*Passiflora incarnata*)
10 g dried wood betony (*Stachys betonica*)
5 g dried lavender flowers (*Lavandula angustifolia*)
water

~ HOW TO MAKE THE TEA ~

1 Mix the herbs and store in a dry, airtight container.

2 Put 2 teaspoons of the mix in a tisane cup and add freshly boiled water. Steep for 5–10 minutes. Strain.

DOSAGE *Drink a cup about 30 minutes before going to bed. If required, make another cup and store in a vacuum flask to drink during the night.*

Supplementary treatments

■ Add 5 drops of lavender oil, or 500 ml chamomile infusion (to make, see p. 84) to the bathwater at night.
■ If overexcitability is causing insomnia, take 2 ml of cowslip flower tincture (to make, see p. 68) in a little warm water before going to bed.

OVER-THE-COUNTER REMEDIES
Mind & Emotions

■ Look for relaxing herbal remedies containing herbs such as chamomile, hops, Jamaican dogwood, pasque flower, passionflower, skullcap, or vervain.
■ Valerian tablets, available from health food stores, can help calm anxiety and sleeplessness.

■ Herbal infusions containing chamomile, linden, or vervain are a valuable supplement to other therapeutic approaches. Use instead of tea and coffee during the day.
■ Bach Flower Remedies are valuable for many different types of emotional problems.

MUSCLES, BONES & JOINTS

HERBAL REMEDIES can relieve the symptoms of creaking joints, aching bones and muscles, as well as treating the cause of the problem and encouraging healing. Long-term aches, such as arthritis, often respond to dietary changes, while cleansing herbal remedies help alleviate the condition by clearing toxins from the system.

Backache & sciatica

Backache is one of the most common reasons for seeking medical help in the West. Finding the cause of the problem is important, since mechanical damage affecting disks or pinched nerves (as in sciatica) can often be helped by osteopathy or chiropractic treatments. Massage can help relieve aching muscles.

Fresh lavender flowers

Lavender oil

LAVENDER *is a mild local analgesic. It relieves aches and pains and encourages relaxation.*

—— *LAVENDER & THYME RUB* ——

Lavender oil is a mild analgesic and can relieve many types of backache, while thyme is an antispasmodic that relaxes overtense muscles. They can be combined with warming oils to soothe aches and pains.

~ INGREDIENTS ~
10 drops lavender oil
(*Lavandula angustifolia*)
10 drops thyme oil (*Thymus vulgaris*)
5 drops juniper oil (*Juniperus communis*)
10 drops eucalyptus oil (*Eucalyptus globulus*)
5 drops pine oil (*Pinus sylvestris*)
18 ml infused St.-John's-wort oil
(*Hypericum perforatum*)

Fresh thyme aerial parts

Thyme oil

THYME *is stimulating and antispasmodic, helping to ease muscle aches and pains.*

Fresh juniper twigs & berries

~ HOW TO MAKE THE RUB ~
Take care to use good quality oils (see p. 83). To make the infused St.-John's-wort oil, see p. 73. Mix the oils in a 100 ml sterilized, dark glass bottle and shake well.

APPLICATION *Pour about a teaspoonful of the oil onto one palm and gently rub your hands together before massaging into painful areas. Repeat at least twice a day.*

JUNIPER *is mildly analgesic and increases blood flow to the skin, encouraging healing.*

Juniper oil

Fresh eucalpytus leaves

EUCALYPTUS *helps to encourage blood flow to the surface, and is effective for aches and pains.*

Eucalyptus oil

SUPPLEMENTARY TREATMENTS

■ A compress (see p. 71) soaked in 15 ml cramp bark tincture and 5 ml cinnamon tincture diluted in 100 ml hot water can help relieve backache. (To make the tinctures, see p. 68.)

■ Mix 2 ml each St.-John's-wort, cramp bark, and willow bark tinctures and dilute with a little warm water. Sip 3 times a day.

■ For chronic conditions, drinking an infusion of St.-John's-wort and valerian (to make, see p. 64) can help.

■ Consult a doctor if the pain starts with an accidental injury. Take homeopathic *Arnica* 6x tablets and repeat at hourly intervals for up to 12 hours to ease shock and trauma.

CAUTIONS FOR BACKACHE

• *Massage is not an appropriate treatment for inflammation or where there is any kind of injury. If in doubt always get professional advice.*

• *Painful areas shouldbe massaged gently.*

• *If sudden back pain does not clear within a few days, seek professional assistance.*

Pine oil

PINE *is a traditional remedy for sciatica. It eases muscle pain and is a stimulant, helping to counteract fatigue.*

Fresh pine twigs

LAVENDER & THYME RUB relaxes tense muscles and relieves pain. It is ideal for soothing backache. Stored in a dark glass bottle, it will keep for at least 3 months.

Lavender & thyme rub

ST.-JOHN'S-WORT *is anti-inflammatory, helping to repair damaged tissues and ease pain.*

Fresh St.-John's-wort flowers

Infused St.-John's-wort oil

Rheumatism

Also known as lumbago or fibrositis, muscular rheumatism (*myalgia*) is common from late middle age onward. In this condition, the connective tissues and tendons associated with leg or arm muscles become inflamed. Warming rubs can often help to relieve the discomfort, and internal remedies are also useful when the condition is persistent.

—— BOGBEAN & MEADOWSWEET TEA ——

Bogbean is a wild water plant, often found in bogs and shallow ponds. Meadowsweet, also, likes to grow in damp ditches and hedgerows. Both are anti-inflammatory and digestive stimulants. By stimulating and strengthening the digestion, the herbs help clear the buildup of toxins that are frequently associated with muscle and joint disorders. They have a bitter taste, disguised in this remedy with licorice extract.

~ INGREDIENTS ~
15 g dried bogbean leaves (*Menyanthes trifoliata*)
10 g dried meadowsweet (*Filipendula ulmaria*)
5 g dried yarrow (*Achillea millefolium*)
5 ml licorice fluid extract (*Glycyrrhiza glabra*)
500 ml water

~ HOW TO MAKE THE TEA ~
1 Mix the dried herbs together in a teapot or jug and pour on freshly boiled water. Steep for 10 minutes and strain.

2 Add the licorice extract to the strained infusion and stir well. Store in a covered jug in a cool place.

DOSAGE *Take a wineglass dose 3 times a day, reheating each time.*

Supplementary treatments
■ Use a rub made from 10 drops each of lavender, marjoram, thyme, and juniper oil in 20 ml of sweet almond oil on aching areas several times a day.
■ If pain prevents sleep, take 5 ml each of wild lettuce tincture, and passionflower tincture in some warm water before going to bed (to make the tinctures, see p. 68).
■ Warm compresses can sometimes help: mix 10 ml arnica tincture, 20 ml cramp bark tincture, and 20 ml angelica root tincture in 150 ml of hot water (to make the tinctures, see p. 68). Soak a pad in the the solution and apply to the painful area. Reheat the mixture for a fresh compress.
Caution: Do not use arnica on broken skin.

Cramps

Muscle cramps can be related to poor circulation and varicose veins, as well as stress, fatigue, and mineral imbalance. They are also common during pregnancy. Sudden cramps in hot weather can be a sign of salt deficiency.

—— CRAMP BARK & LAVENDER RUB ——

Another name for cramp bark is guelder rose. Cramp bark's name accurately describes its relaxing action. This rub is suitable for all kinds of muscle cramps.

~ INGREDIENTS ~
25 ml cramp bark tincture (*Viburnum opulus*)
2 ml lavender oil (*Lavandula angustifolia*)
2 ml marjoram oil (*Origanum vulgare*)
20 ml sweet almond oil

~ HOW TO MAKE THE RUB ~
To make the tincture, see p. 68. Mix the ingredients in a 50 ml sterilized, dark glass bottle and shake thoroughly.

APPLICATION *Apply a little of the rub to the affected area, and massage vigorously. Repeat, as required, shaking the bottle thoroughly each time.*

Frozen shoulder & tennis elbow

Frozen shoulder is a chronic stiffness of the shoulder joint, and tennis elbow is inflammation of the tendons on the outside of the elbow joint.

—— YARROW & ST.-JOHN'S-WORT RUB ——

Yarrow and St.-John's-wort are anti-inflammatory. They are used to help ease muscle tension.

~ INGREDIENTS ~
2.5 ml yarrow oil (*Achillea millefolium*)
2.5 ml lavender oil (*Lavandula angustifolia*)
20 ml infused St.-John's-wort oil (*Hypericum perforatum*)

~ HOW TO MAKE THE RUB ~
To make the infused oil, see p. 73. Mix the oils in a 25 ml sterilized, dark glass bottle and shake well.

APPLICATION *Put a little on your fingers and massage well into aching elbows or stiff shoulders. Repeat 3 or 4 times a day.*

Gout

The painful, swollen joints of gout are caused by a buildup of uric acid crystals in the tissues. Rich food, too much alcohol, and excessive amounts of shellfish or fatty fish can all exacerbate the problem and should be avoided. Cutting out caffeine and giving up smoking can also help.

CELERY & HEATHER TEA

Successful treatment of gout requires diuretics, which help the condition by clearing excess uric acid from the system. Celery seed, heather flowers, and yarrow all have effective diuretic actions.

~ INGREDIENTS ~

50 g dried celery seed (*Apium graveolens*)
15 g dried heather flowers (*Calluna vulgaris*)
15 g dried yarrow (*Achillea millefolium*)
250 ml water

~ HOW TO MAKE THE TEA ~

1 Mix the herbs and store in a dry, airtight container.

2 Put 2 teaspoons of the mix in a jug or teapot and add freshly boiled water. Steep for 10 minutes and strain.

DOSAGE *Drink half while still warm. Reheat and take the other half later in the day. Make a fresh tea each day.*

Supplementary treatments

- If the sufferer can bear it, a poultice of mashed cabbage leaf placed gently on the affected area can help. To make the poultice, see p. 71.
- Eat plenty of asparagus, which is a good diuretic.
- Devil's claw is an effective anti-inflammatory and may be useful. Take 2 x 200 mg capsules of the herb 3 to 4 times a day.

Osteoarthritis

Arthritis involves pain and swelling in the joints. It can be caused by general wear-and-tear (osteoarthritis) when usually just one or two joints are affected, or it can be an inflammatory disorder, affecting many joints (rheumatoid arthritis). The latter usually requires complex and extensive professional treatment, but osteoarthritis may respond to home remedies.

ST.-JOHN'S-WORT & CELERY MIX

This combination of tinctures will help to cleanse the system. stimulate the circulation and digestion, and reduce inflammation.

~ INGREDIENTS ~

20 ml St.-John's-wort tincture
(*Hypericum perforatum*)
20 ml celery seed tincture (*Apium graveolens*)
15 ml bogbean tincture (*Menyanthes trifoliata*)
15 ml angelica root tincture (*Angelica archangelica*)
15 ml yellow dock tincture (*Rumex crispus*)
10 ml *Gui Zhi* tincture (*Cinnamomum cassia*)
5 ml licorice tincture (*Glycyrrhiza glabra*)

~ HOW TO MAKE THE MIX ~

To make the individual tinctures, see p. 68. Combine the tinctures in a sterilized, dark glass bottle and shake well.

DOSAGE *Take 5 ml in a little warm water 3 times a day.*

Supplementary treatments

- Take a cup of standard infusion of boneset and yarrow to encourage sweating, thereby helping to clear toxins.
- Rub the affected part several times a day with 5 ml rosemary oil and 5 ml juniper oil in 50 ml infused comfrey oil (to make, see p. 72).

OVER-THE-COUNTER REMEDIES: *Muscles, Bones & Joints*

- Ready-made rubs for muscle, bone, and joint ailments are widely available. Look for mixtures with birch, cajeput, camphor oil and extracts, eucalyptus, juniper, lavender, peppermint, pine, rosemary, thyme, or wintergreen.
- Devil's claw is a potent anti-inflammatory remedy that has become widely available in the past few years. It is either very effective or seems to have no impact at all. Take for at least 6 weeks (following the instructions on

the package) before abandoning the treatment.
- When buying over-the-counter remedies, look for those that contain combinations of angelica, black cohosh, bogbean, burdock, celery seed, lignum vitae resin, meadowsweet, stinging nettles, white willow, yarrow, and yellow dock. These are herbs that cleanse the system, soothe inflammation, and gently stimulate the digestion.

MALE PROBLEMS

IN TRADITIONAL CHINESE medicine, male sexual energy is closely associated with the kidneys, and tonics for this organ are often given to increase fertility and vigor. Problems with the prostate gland are one of the most widespread male disorders; in the West, orthodox treatment usually involves surgery or hormone therapy. Although herbs are no substitute for long-term medication, they provide gentle remedies suitable for mild conditions of both short-term infections and of chronic disorders.

Prostate disorders

The prostate gland sits beneath the bladder. It can become infected and inflamed (a condition known as prostatitis), and is often enlarged in older men, leading to difficulties with urination.

– SAW PALMETTO & SIBERIAN GINSENG MIX –

Saw palmetto has long been used as a sexual tonic. Modern research has confirmed its effectiveness in treating prostate problems – both for inflammation and enlargement. The mix can be used in both cases.

~ INGREDIENTS ~

40 ml saw palmetto tincture (*Serenoa repens*)
35 ml Siberian ginseng tincture
(*Eleutherococcus senticosus*)
25 ml echinacea tincture (*Echinacea angustifolia*)

~ HOW TO MAKE THE MIX ~

To make the individual tinctures, see p. 68. Mix the tinctures together in a 100 ml sterilized, dark glass bottle and shake well.

DOSAGE *Take 5 ml in half a glass of warm water 3 times a day. Increase to 10 ml in acute stages of prostatitis.*

CAUTIONS

• *Medical examination is recommended for prostate disorders because of the risk of prostate cancer.*
• *Do not stop taking long-term medication for prostate problems before first consulting a doctor or professional herbal practitioner.*

Supplementary treatments

■ Make an infusion (see p. 64) using 10 g each of dried white deadnettle, cornsilk, and pellitory-of-the-wall as a healing diuretic tea to help counteract prostate enlargement.
■ Take 500 mg of evening primrose oil daily.

Urethritis

When infections invade the urinary tract the urethra can become inflamed, causing discharge and pain on passing urine. It is important to seek professional medical help, particularly if symptoms are severe. Urethritis can be associated with sexually transmitted diseases, in which case the sufferer will be referred to a specialist clinic. The following remedy and self-help measures can alleviate the symptoms.

— BUCHU & COUCHGRASS TEA —

The South African buchu bush has diuretic and antiseptic properties, and is gently stimulating for the kidneys, while common couchgrass rhizomes provide mucilages to soothe and heal the affected area.

~ INGREDIENTS ~

50 g dried buchu leaves (*Barosma betulina*)
30 g dried couchgrass rhizome (*Agropyron repens*)
20 g dried cornsilk (*Zea mays*)
water

~ HOW TO MAKE THE TEA ~

1 Mix the herbs and store in a dark, airtight container.

2 Put 2 teaspoons of the mix in a tisane cup or small teapot and pour on freshly boiled water. Infuse for 10 minutes and strain.

DOSAGE *Drink a teacup dose up to 6 times a day during the acute stage of infection.*

Supplementary treatments

■ Drink plenty of fluids, adding a pinch of baking soda to each glass of water to help reduce the acid content of the urine. Barleywater can be a particularly soothing drink.
■ Take 2 x 200 mg echinacea capsules 3 times a day.

Infertility

Male infertility is often associated with a low sperm count. Recent Danish research – albeit with only a small sample of men – suggests that modern "junk" foods and high levels of pesticides in food can be contributory factors. Eating organically grown produce, cutting out alcohol, caffeine, and smoking, and wearing loose clothing can all help.

—— *He Shou Wu & cinnamon wine* ——

He Shou Wu, or "fleeceflower," has been used as a reproductive energy tonic by the Chinese for generations. Taoist sages reputedly lived for centuries by taking the herb, and it is traditionally used to increase sperm count.

~ Ingredients ~
250 g dried *He Shou Wu* (*Polygonum multiflorum*)
150 g dried cinnamon bark (*Cinnamomum zeylanicum*)
100 g dried licorice root (*Glycyrrhiza glabra*)
1–2 liters red wine

~ How to make the wine ~

1 Put all the herbs into a large vinegar vat, or similar crockery pot.

2 Pour on the red wine to fill the pot and cover the herbs completely.

3 Leave the mixture to steep for 10–14 days.

Dosage *Take a sherry glass dose of the mixture daily, adding more red wine to keep the herbs covered.*

Note: The mixture will last for several months if it is kept well covered with wine. Discard if there is any sign of mold on the herbs.

Supplementary treatments
■ Take 2 garlic pearls and 500 mg ginseng capsules daily.
■ Ensure adequate intake of vitamins B-complex and E and keep zinc levels up by eating pumpkin seeds regularly.
■ If stress may be contributing to the problem, take skullcap, vervain, linden, or chamomile infusions (see p. 64).

Impotence

Stress, exhaustion, and excessive alcohol can all contribute to sexual problems, with low libido and difficulties with intercourse. Herbs have been used as aphrodisiacs in all cultures for centuries, and both Chinese and Ayurvedic medicine make a contribution with herbs such as *Wu Wei Zi* (schizandra berries) and *ashwagandha* (withania roots), which may be found in patent remedies.

—— *Damiana & cinnamon tea* ——

Damiana was traditionally used in tropical America as a potent aphrodisiac – indeed, its botanical name was once Turnera aphrodisiaca. Schizandra has been used for centuries in China as a sexual tonic suitable for both men and women, enhancing staying power and vigor.

~ Ingredients ~
10 g dried cinnamon bark (*Cinnamomum zeylanicum*)
10 g *Wu Wei Zi* (dried schizandra berries – *Schisandra chinensis*)
15 g dried damiana leaf (*Turnera diffusa*)
500 ml water

~ How to make the tea ~

1 Mix the cinnamon, *Wu Wei Zi*, and water in a pan and simmer for 15 minutes to make a decoction.

2 Put the damiana leaf in a teapot and pour on the simmering decoction.

3 Steep for a further 10 minutes and strain well. Store in a covered jug in a cool place.

Dosage *Drink a wineglass dose 3 times a day before meals.*

Supplementary treatments
■ Try body massage with essential oils before intercourse – jasmine, ylang ylang, rose, patchouli, and sandalwood all have an aphrodisiac effect. Use 5 drops of essential oil of any of these in 5 ml of sweet almond oil.

OVER-THE-COUNTER REMEDIES *Male Problems*

■ Herbal aphrodisiacs come in all shapes and sizes – not all efficacious or containing even remotely suitable herbs. Look for remedies that include: *Bu Gu Zhi* (psoralea berries), damiana, *Dang Gui* (Chinese angelica), ginseng, *He Shou Wu* (fleeceflower root), and saw palmetto.

■ Herbal diuretics and urinary antiseptics are widely available in blends or tea bags. Look for those containing bearberry, buchu, celery seed, cleavers, cornsilk, couchgrass, dandelion, and yarrow. Avoid long-term use of diuretics containing juniper, which can irritate the kidneys.

FEMALE PROBLEMS

OLD HERBALS ARE FULL OF remedies for gynecological problems –
many of them concerned with improving fertility, regulating periods,
or easing childbirth (a life-threatening situation in bygone days).
Today, Western medicine tends to blame hormonal deficiencies
for many disorders, while the Chinese focus on energy imbalance
in organs associated with the female reproductive system,
and treat menstrual problems with liver tonics and
menopausal disorders with kidney remedies.

Heavy periods

Excessive bleeding is a common menstrual problem. It is
important to consult a doctor or professional herbalist to ensure
that no significant causes – such as fibroids or
endometriosis – are involved. Heavy bleeding often
leads to anemia, so eat plenty of iron-rich foods.

*Fresh lady's
mantle aerial
parts*

LADY'S MANTLE,
*as its name suggests, is a
traditional women's remedy.
It is widely
used in Europe.*

LADY'S MANTLE & SHEPHERD'S PURSE TEA

*Lady's mantle, like other members of the rose
family, is a good astringent. It also helps regulate
menstrual imbalances. Shepherd's purse – also known as
"mother's hearts" – is useful for reducing excess bleeding.*

~ INGREDIENTS ~

20 g dried lady's mantle (*Alchemilla vulgaris*)
10 g dried shepherd's purse (*Capsella bursa-pastoris*)
10 g dried raspberry leaves (*Rubus idaeus*)
5 g dried pot marigold petals (*Calendula officinalis*)
5 g dried mugwort leaves (*Artemisia vulgaris*)
500 ml water

*Dried lady's
mantle aerial
parts*

*Fresh
shepherd's
purse aerial
parts*

~ HOW TO MAKE THE TEA ~

1 Mix the dried herbs together. Reserve one half
for the following day, storing it in a dry, airtight
container. Place the other half in a teapot or jug.

2 Add the freshly boiled water.

3 Steep for 10 minutes and strain. Store the surplus in a
covered jug in a cool place.

DOSAGE *The tea may be taken for a few months as a preventative
measure. Drink a teacup dose 3 times a day, reheating if preferred.*

*Dried shepherd's
purse aerial parts*

SHEPHERD'S PURSE *is highly
valued in both Eastern and
Western herbal repertoires for
its astringent properties.*

RASPBERRY LEAVES *are best known in remedies to prepare mothers for childbirth, but their astringent quality also makes them useful for treating heavy periods.*

Fresh raspberry leaves

Dried raspberry leaves

Fresh pot marigold

Dried pot marigold petals

POT MARIGOLD *acts as a menstrual regulator, restoring the normal cycle. It stimulates the liver and is also astringent.*

LADY'S MANTLE & SHEPHERD'S PURSE TEA is a gentle herbal remedy for recurring heavy periods with no obvious cause. It helps normalize the menstrual cycle and regulate the blood flow.

Dried mugwort leaves

Fresh mugwort aerial parts

MUGWORT *is a nervine. It stimulates the uterus and regulates the menstrual cycle.*

Lady's mantle & shepherd's purse tea

Premenstrual syndrome

Western medicine usually describes premenstrual syndrome (PMS) in terms of hormonal imbalance, while Asian theories define it in terms of energy imbalance or stagnation. Typical symptoms include emotional upsets, irritability, breast tenderness, food cravings, and digestive irregularities. Symptoms ease when menstruation starts. Relaxation and avoiding stimulants, such as caffeine, can help.

—— DANG GUI & PEONY DECOCTION ——

This is based on a classical Chinese formula called "free and easy," which is often given to relieve the energy blocks contributing to PMS. Most of the herbs act on the liver, an organ associated with the female reproductive system.

~ INGREDIENTS ~

20 g *Dang Gui* (Chinese angelica – *Angelica sinensis*)
20 g *Bai Shao* (white peony root – *Paeonia lactiflora*)
5 g *Chen Pi* (dried tangerine peel – *Citrus reticulata*)
5 g dried licorice root (*Glycyrrhiza glabra*)
2 g fresh ginger root (*Zingiber officinalis*)
10 g dried vervain (*Verbena officinalis*)
2 g dried peppermint (*Mentha piperita*)
1 liter water

~ HOW TO MAKE THE DECOCTION ~

1 Simmer the *Dang Gui*, *Bai Shao*, *Chen Pi*, licorice and ginger roots, and water in a pan for 15–20 minutes.

2 Put the vervain and peppermint into a teapot. Strain the simmering decoction onto the herbs. Steep for 10 minutes, strain into a jug, and store in a cool place.

DOSAGE *The tea may be taken for a few months as a preventative measure. Drink a wineglass dose up to 5 times a day.*

Supplementary treatments

■ Take 10–20 drops of chaste-tree berry tincture each morning before breakfast (to make the tincture, see p. 68).
■ To ensure adequate intake of essential fatty acids, take 1 g daily of evening primrose or borage oils.

Period pain

There are various types of period pain: cramps when menstruation starts; the feeling of heaviness beforehand; and spasmodic aches before bleeding. In many cases exercise can relieve period pain, and a brisk walk is often more beneficial than curling up with a hotwater bottle. Relaxation, a healthy sex life, and avoiding stimulants, such as caffeine, may also help.

—— BLACK HAW TINCTURE ——

One of the best remedies for period cramps is black haw bark – a relaxing herb that has a specific action on the uterus. It works very well when taken on its own, but here it is combined with St.-John's-wort, a restorative nerve tonic and pasque flower, which has antispasmodic properties.

~ INGREDIENTS ~

15 ml black haw bark tincture (*Viburnum prunifolium*)
2.5 ml St.-John's-wort tincture (*Hypericum perforatum*)
2.5 ml pasque flower tincture (*Anemone vulgaris*)

~ HOW TO MAKE THE TINCTURE ~

To make the individual tinctures, see p. 68. Combine the tinctures in a sterilized, dark glass bottle.

DOSAGE *Take the whole quantity in a tumbler of warm water when period cramps start. Repeat up to 3 times a day as required.*

Supplementary treatments

■ To encourage relaxation, drink an infusion made from equal parts of dried St.-John's-wort, raspberry leaves, and skullcap (to make the infusion, see p. 64).
■ Dilute 10 drops each of cypress, marjoram, and rosemary oil in 20 ml of sweet almond oil and gently massage into the abdomen.

Ingredients for Dang Gui & peony decoction

Fresh vervain

Dang Gui

Bai Shao

Chen Pi

Fresh peppermint

Dried licorice root

Fresh ginger root

*Red clover &
nettle tea*

Red clover

Nettle

Infertility

The struggle to conceive can become a full-time preoccupation for many people. Modern fertilization techniques have done much to help. Herbs can improve general health and readiness for conception but in general, they should be seen as supporting other approaches, rather than a remedy in themselves.

——— RED CLOVER & NETTLE TEA ———

Red clover is a good cleansing remedy, reputedly containing estrogen-like compounds, while nettles are nourishing for the whole body. Peppermint is a good sexual stimulant and marigold strengthens the reproductive organs.

~ INGREDIENTS ~

45 g dried red clover flowers (*Trifolium pratense*)
25 g dried stinging nettle (*Urtica dioica*)
10 g dried peppermint (*Mentha piperita*)
20 g dried pot marigold petals (*Calendula officinalis*)
water

~ HOW TO MAKE THE TEA ~

1 Mix the herbs and store in an airtight, dark jar.

2 Place 2 teaspoons in a tisane cup or small teapot and add a cup of freshly boiled water. Steep for 10 minutes and strain.

DOSAGE *Drink a teacup dose 2 or 3 times a day.*

Supplementary treatments

■ Take 5 drops of false unicorn tincture daily in a little warm water (to make the tincture, see p. 68).
■ Look for patent remedies based on *Dang Gui,* a herb that stimulates the reproductive system.
■ Chronic low-grade infections such as recurring candida or cystitis can affect fertility. Take remedies suggested for these conditions (see pp. 124 & 127) and boost the immune system by taking a 200 mg echinacea capsule 3 times a day.

Menopause

As women age, hormonal levels fall, until there are insufficient amounts to trigger the usual monthly menstruation, at which point ovulation and regular periods come to an end. Hormone levels continue to wax and wane, however, and menopausal women may continue to experience symptoms similar to premenstrual syndrome. Menopausal problems can include hot flashes, night sweats, palpitations, vaginal dryness, sore eyes, and emotional upsets.

——— HE SHOU WU & VERVAIN MIX ———

In Chinese tradition, menopausal problems are associated with run-down kidney energies, so tonics such as He Shou Wu that act on those organs are prescribed. Vervain is a good liver tonic and sedative to calm emotional upsets, while sage and wild yam help with more symptomatic menopausal problems.

~ INGREDIENTS ~

30 ml *He Shou Wu* tincture (fleeceflower root – *Polygonum multiflorum*)
20 ml vervain tincture (*Verbena officinalis*)
20 ml sage tincture (*Salvia officinalis*)
15 ml wild yam root tincture (*Dioscorea villosa*)
10 ml lavender tincture (*Lavandula angustifolia*)
5 ml licorice tincture (*Glycyrrhiza glabra*)

~ HOW TO MAKE THE MIX ~

To make the individual tinctures, see p. 68. Mix the tinctures and store in a 100 ml sterilized, dark glass bottle.

DOSAGE *Take 5 ml in a tumbler of warm water 3 times a day before meals.*

Supplementary treatments

■ If palpitations are a problem, make an infusion with 10 g each of dried motherwort, hawthorn tops, and mugwort to 500 ml freshly boiled water (to make the infusion, see p. 64). Take a wineglass dose 3 times a day.
■ Apply vitamin E oil directly to the vagina to ease dryness. Regular sexual intercourse will help maintain a healthy vaginal lining.
■ For hot flashes and night sweats, make an infusion with 15 g each of dried sage and dried mugwort to 500 ml freshly boiled water (to make the infusion, see p. 64). Take a wineglass dose 3 times a day. Alternatively, take a 200 mg goldenseal capsule 2 or 3 times a day for acute cases (to make the capsules, see p. 70).

Loss of libido

As with men, loss of sexual desire can be caused by a number of factors including exhaustion, stress, and an excess of stimulants such as caffeine. The rhythm of the menstrual cycle also plays a part, with libido often rising in midcycle, falling, and rising again just before bleeding starts. Stimulating herbal tonics can often help to counter loss of libido; learning to relax is also very important.

RASPBERRY & ROSEMARY TEA

As well as herbs that have a specific reputation as aphrodisiacs, sexual energies can be generally improved with nourishing, stimulating herbs. Nettle is rich in minerals and vitamins, rosemary is stimulating, and raspberry leaves help to relax the reproductive organs.

~ INGREDIENTS ~
40 g dried raspberry leaves (*Rubus idaeus*)
20 g dried stinging nettles (*Urtica dioica*)
15 g dried rosemary (*Rosmarinus officinalis*)
15 g dried chaste-tree berries (*Vitex agnus-castus*)
10 g dried peppermint (*Mentha piperita*)
water

~ HOW TO MAKE THE TEA ~
1 Mix the herbs and store in an airtight, dark jar.

2 Place 2 teaspoons of the mixture in a tisane cup or small teapot. Add a cup of freshly boiled water and steep for 10 minutes. Strain.

DOSAGE *Drink a teacup 2 or 3 times a day.*

Supplementary treatments
■ Chaste-tree can raise women's hormonal activity and enhance sexuality. In addition to the tea, take 10–20 drops of tincture (to make, see p. 68) in warm water before breakfast.
■ Use essential oils in massage before intercourse – try 5–10 drops of jasmine, sandalwood, rose, ylang ylang, clary, or neroli in 10 ml of sweet almond oil.
■ Drink a sherry glass daily of tonic wine made with *Wu Wei Zi* (schizandra berries). To make, see p. 69.
■ Relaxing herbs can help if tension is a problem. Make a standard infusion (see p. 64) using equal parts of skullcap, vervain, and wood betony.
■ Stimulating herbs can improve vitality. Take 5–10 drops of ginger or cinnamon tinctures in warm water daily.

Vaginal infections

Vaginal secretions and the friendly bacteria they harbor usually prevent infections from taking hold, but the quality of vaginal secretions can change as a result of factors such as taking contraceptive pills, stress, general infections, antibiotic treatments, or food intolerance. These give rise to conditions in which vaginal infections can develop. Candida, a fungal infection characterized by a white discharge and itching, is one of the most common problems.

POT MARIGOLD & TEA TREE PESSARIES

Pot marigold is a useful antifungal and tea tree is one of the most effective herbal antiseptics available.

~ INGREDIENTS ~
20 g cocoa butter
10 drops pot marigold oil (*Calendula officinalis*)
10 drops tea tree oil (*Melaleuca alternifolia*)
5 drops thyme oil (*Thymus vulgaris*)

~ HOW TO MAKE THE PESSARIES ~
1 Melt the cocoa butter in a double boiler or a bowl over hot water.

2 Make and lubricate foil shapes or a pessary mold as described on p. 70.

3 Remove the cocoa butter from the heat and add the oils. Stir well and pour into the pessary mold or foil shapes. Allow to set. (This takes about 4 hours.) Remove from the mold or foil shapes. Store in a cool place in an airtight jar or pot lined with waxed paper.

APPLICATION *Insert a pessary into the vagina at night and repeat in the morning while the infection persists.*

OVER-THE-COUNTER REMEDIES
Female Problems

■ Look for patent remedies containing *Bai Shao* (white peony) or *Dang Gui* (Chinese angelica), which can ease many menstrual disorders.
■ Evening primrose oil or other oils that are rich in essential fatty acids (e.g. borage, walnut, linseed, or black currant) can help menstrual problems.
■ For menopausal problems, remedies based on blue cohosh, *Dang Gui*, false unicorn root, goldenseal, *He Shou Wu*, *Nu Zhen Zi*, or sage, may be helpful.
■ Chaste-tree berry tablets are useful for many disorders.

PREGNANCY & CHILDBIRTH

HERBAL REMEDIES HAVE been used by generations of women to ease problems associated with pregnancy and childbirth. Many provide a safe alternative to orthodox remedies, but should still be used with respect during pregnancy. See the general caution on p. 126. There are herbal remedies available for common ailments that are particularly suitable for pregnant women. These include American ginseng as an energy tonic, butternut for constipation, and nettle tea for anemia (see pp. 104 and 109).

Morning sickness

Nausea and vomiting is common in early pregnancy, beginning in the third or fourth week and lasting up to three months. Occasionally they persist throughout pregnancy, and sufferers may need hospital treatment. Sufferers should consult a doctor if sickness is severe.

SIMPLE TINCTURES

Placing a few drops of tincture on the tongue is often the best way to take remedies when feeling nauseous.

~ TINCTURES ~
10 ml ginger tincture (*Zingiber officinalis*)
10 ml chamomile tincture (*Matricaria recutita*)
10 ml *Chen Pi* tincture (*Citrus reticulata*)
10 ml black horehound tincture (*Ballota nigra*)
10 ml peppermint tincture (*Mentha piperita*)
10 ml fennel seed tincture (*Foeniculum officinalis*)

~ HOW TO TAKE THE TINCTURES ~
To make the tinctures see p. 68. Put each one into a separate 10 ml sterilized, dark glass dropper bottle.

DOSAGE *Place 2–3 drops of the chosen tincture on the tongue at the first sign of nausea. There is no simple rule for treating morning sickness and sufferers should experiment to discover which tincture suits them best, and vary the remedies as required.*

Supplementary treatments
■ Morning sickness can be related to digestive problems. Take 1–2 x 200 mg slippery elm capsules daily.
■ To encourage relaxation, sip an infusion (to make, see p. 64) of 35 g dried lemon balm, 15 g dried skullcap, 10 g dried lavender, and 10 g dried peppermint, in teacup doses.
■ Ginger is very effective for morning sickness. Take 1 g per day in capsule form, or chew crystallized ginger.

Fluid retention (edema)

Swollen ankles and puffiness of the hands or face are common problems in pregnancy. The growing baby sometimes upsets the protein balance of the blood, causing expectant mothers to retain as much as 5–6 liters of fluid. Simple edema can be relieved with rest, eating grapes, asparagus, and apples, limiting salt intake, and the use of gentle diuretic teas to encourage elimination of excess fluid.

CORNSILK & DANDELION TEA

This simple diuretic herbal remedy can help cut down excess fluid in the system. Dandelion leaves are rich in potassium while cornsilk is soothing for the urinary tract.

~ INGREDIENTS ~
50 g dried dandelion leaves (*Taraxacum officinale*)
30 g dried cornsilk (*Zea mays*)
20 g dried couchgrass rhizome (*Agropyron repens*)
water

~ HOW TO MAKE THE TEA ~
1 Mix the herbs and store in an airtight jar.

2 Place 2 teaspoons of the mixture in a tisane cup or small teapot. Add a cup of freshly boiled water and steep for 10 minutes. Strain.

DOSAGE *Drink a cup 2 or 3 times a day while symptoms persist.*

CAUTION
• *Protein in the urine can be an indication that toxemia is developing – other symptoms include headaches and raised blood pressure. If swelling in the ankles is not relieved by rest or is "pitting" (finger pressure leaves significant indentations in the flesh), seek professional medical help quickly.*

Preparing for childbirth

For centuries, women have taken herbs to prepare for an easy delivery, to ease labor pains and ultimately, to help clear the placenta. Today modern medicine provides a battery of more sophisticated options but, for uncomplicated births, herbs still have an important role. About six weeks before the baby is due start preparing with a daily cup of raspberry leaf tea (to make, see p. 64). Once labor starts, take Wood Betony & Rose Petal Tea.

—— WOOD BETONY & ROSE PETAL TEA ——

Wood betony helps to soothe the nervous system and ease tensions as well as stimulate uterine contractions. Rose petals are very uplifting – both physically and spiritually.

~ INGREDIENTS ~

50 g dried wood betony (*Stachys betonica*)
20 g dried rose petals (*Rosa gallica* or *R. centifolia*)
20 g dried raspberry leaves (*Rubus idaeus*)
10 g cinnamon stick (*Cinnamomum zeylanicum*)
500 ml water

~ HOW TO MAKE THE TEA ~

1. Mix the herbs and store in am airtight, dark jar.

2. Put one-third into a teapot and pour on the freshly boiled water. Steep for 10 minutes. Strain.

DOSAGE *Sip a mugful during labor. Repeat as often as required.*

Note: In the final stages of labor add 10 g dried basil leaves to the herbal mixture and infuse as before.

Supplementary treatments

■ Once labor starts, massage the abdomen regularly with 10 drops each of clove and sage oil and 3 drops of rose oil in 10 ml of sweet almond oil.
■ Place a hot compress soaked in pot marigold infusion to which 2–3 drops of sage oil have been added, across the lower abdomen above the pubic area. Replace as the compress cools. (To make the compress, see p. 71.)
■ Take homeopathic *Arnica* 6x tablets every 15–20 minutes after the birth for 2–4 hours to help recovery.

OTHER PROBLEMS IN PREGNANCY

See also: anemia, p. 109; backache, p. 114; constipation, p. 104; cramps, p. 116; cystitis 117; hemorrhoids (piles), p. 106; high blood pressure, p. 108; indigestion & heartburn, p. 107; insomnia, p. 113; vaginal infections, p. 124; varicose veins, p. 109.

Breastfeeding problems

Most child care experts acknowledge that "breast is best" for feeding a newborn baby, but establishing a relaxed pattern of breastfeeding can be difficult for many new mothers.

1. Increasing milk flow

Herbs may be used to encourage milk flow, and frequent feedings are also important. Mix together 20 g fennel seeds, 30 g dried goat's rue, 30 g dried vervain, 20 g dried stinging nettles, and a teaspoon of powdered cinnamon. Store the mix in an airtight jar. Take a single cup infusion (to make, see p. 64) 4 times a day. In addition, take 5 drops of chaste-tree berry tincture in warm water before breakfast, and avoid spicy foods as the flavors will often permeate the milk supply.

2. Sore nipples

Cracked and sore nipples can be a deterrent to breastfeeding and can lead to engorgement. Apply calendula cream (available over the counter) or a little honey mixed with sweet almond oil to the nipples at frequent intervals.

3. Engorgement & mastitis

If milk remains in the breast at the end of feedings they may become engorged and painful; if ducts become blocked, inflammation and infection – mastitis – may follow. A simple but effective herbal remedy for engorgement and mastitis is to place a cabbage leaf (thoroughly washed and softened by beating with a cooking mallet) inside the bra.

GENERAL CAUTIONS FOR PREGNANCY

• *Do not take alcoholic tinctures or tonic wines during pregnancy.*
• *Many herbs should be avoided in pregnancy. If in doubt, seek professional advice. In the first 3 months, avoid medication and do not use the following herbs at all during pregnancy: arbor vitae, barberry, basil oil, black cohosh, blue cohosh, chamomile oil, Dang Gui, feverfew, goldenseal, greater celandine, juniper, lady's mantle, mistletoe, motherwort, mugwort, myrrh, pennyroyal, pokeroot, rue, shepherd's purse, southernwood,tansy, and wormwood. Do not take large or therapeutic doses of the following during pregnancy: angelica, bitter orange, cayenne, celery seed, cinnamon, cowslip, elder bark, fennel, fenugreek, ginseng, lavender, marjoram, nutmeg, parsley, rhubarb root, senna, sage, tea, thyme, vervain, wild yam, wood betony, and yarrow.*

URINARY TRACT PROBLEMS

REPEATED URINARY TRACT PROBLEMS can be a sign of energy weakness or immune deficiency. Recurrent cystitis, for example, can be related to thrush, which often arises when the immune system is under stress. In Chinese medicine, kidney energy is linked to reproduction and creativity, and can be easily worn down by childbearing or overwork, leading to urinary problems. Some herbs are useful urinary antiseptics and help to clear infections, while others are warming and energizing, helping the system heal itself.

Cystitis

Cystitis is inflammation of the bladder and tends to be more common in women. The symptoms usually include cloudy, unpleasant-smelling urine, frequent urination, a burning sensation on passing water, and low groin pain. It can be a recurrent problem, and may be triggered by bacteria passing into the urinary tract from fecal material or during intercourse.

— *MARSHMALLOW & CORNSILK MIXTURE* —

Marshmallow is rich in mucilages to ease inflamed membranes, while yarrow is astringent and healing.

~ INGREDIENTS ~
30 ml marshmallow tincture (*Althaea officinalis*)
30 ml bearberry tincture (*Arctostaphylos uva-ursi*)
20 ml cornsilk tincture (*Zea mays*)
10 ml couchgrass tincture (*Agropyron repens*)
10 ml yarrow tincture (*Achillea millefolium*)

~ HOW TO MAKE THE MIXTURE ~
To make the individual tinctures see p. 68. Mix the tinctures together in a 100 ml sterilized, dark glass bottle.

DOSAGE *Put 5 ml in a glass and pour on some boiling water. Allow to cool, then sip. Take 4 times a day.*

CAUTION
• *Seek professional medical help if symptoms do not ease after a few days or if there are signs of kidney involvement (fever and loin pain).*

Supplementary treatments
■ Take the tea recommended for urethritis on p. 118.
■ Take 2 x 200 mg capsules of echinacea 3 times a day to fight infections. Drink plenty of water and avoid alcohol.

CAUTION FOR KIDNEY PROBLEMS
• *Kidney infections require professional treatment. Seek medical help if a bladder or urinary tract infection is accompanied by loin pain or feverishness. Kidney stones should always be referred to a professional practitioner.*

Kidney stones

Kidney stones are formed from deposits of uric acid or calcium salts crystallizing in highly concentrated urine and collecting in the urinary tract. The urine usually appears cloudy and passing water may feel uncomfortable and "gritty."

— *PELLITORY & GRAVELROOT TEA* —

Both pellitory-of-the-wall and gravelroot are effective at breaking up and encouraging elimination of kidney stones. Pellitory is a Mediterranean relative of the stinging nettle, while gravelroot originates from the US.

~ INGREDIENTS ~
15 g dried gravelroot (*Eupatorium purpureum*)
10 g dried marshmallow root (*Althaea officinalis*)
10 g dried pellitory-of-the-wall (*Parietaria diffusa*)
10 g celery seed (*Apium graveolens*)
5 g dried cornsilk (*Zea mays*)
750 ml water

~ HOW TO MAKE THE TEA ~
1 Put the gravelroot, marshmallow, and water in a pan and simmer for 15–20 minutes to make a decoction.

2 Place the other herbs in a teapot or jug and pour the simmering decoction over them. Infuse for 10 minutes. Strain into a jug. Cover and store in a cool place.

DOSAGE *Drink a mugful 4 times a day.*

CHILDREN'S COMPLAINTS

MANY CHILDREN'S AILMENTS are mild and self-limiting, although symptoms can be dramatic, with sudden fevers and soaring temperatures. Home treatment is often sufficient, although it is important to seek medical help urgently if symptoms are acute or of increasing severity. Herbs provide gentle remedies that are safe even for young babies.

CAUTION

Some remedies can taste bitter and may need to be sweetened with fruit juice or honey. Give children under a year old only pasteurized honey or honey that has been boiled for 5 minutes.

DOSAGE FOR BABIES & CHILDREN

All doses given in this section are suitable for babies and children. If using remedies elsewhere in the book for children, remember to reduce the dose accordingly. For children under 2 years, use a fifth of the adult dose, increasing gradually to reach a quarter of the adult dose at 3 or 4 (depending on the size of the child), a third at 6 or 7, a half at 8 or 9, and then increasing to the full adult dose at puberty.

Babies: Sleeplessness

Sleepless babies soon make the rest of the household tense and irritable, compounding the problem. Make sure the room is not too hot, the baby is comfortable, feels safe and secure, and is not hungry or thirsty. Give lots of cuddles.

--- CHAMOMILE BATH ---

Chamomile is one of the best herbs for small babies: sedative and calming for the digestive system, it is ideal for soothing overexcitement which can contribute to sleeplessness.

~ INGREDIENTS ~
2 drops chamomile oil (*Matricaria recutita*)
1 drop lavender oil (*Lavandula angustifolia*)

~ HOW TO USE THE MIXTURE ~
Add the oils to the bath and agitate the water well before bathing the baby.

Supplementary treatments
■ Gentle massage can help calm small babies – stroke forearms repeatedly rather than trying body massage. Use a single drop of chamomile oil in 20 ml of sweet almond oil.
■ Avoid caffeine if breastfeeding. If the child is eating solids, check foods for artificial colorants or additives and ensure adequate intake of vitamins and minerals.
■ Give 25–50 ml infusion at night (to make, see p. 64) using 10 g of dried chamomile flowers, catnip, wood betony or lemon balm to 500 ml water.

Babies: Diaper rash

Diaper rash is a common affliction and can be very painful and irritating. It can be caused by irregular or inefficient diaper changes and it can also be related to digestive problems and yeast infections, so it is important to check the diet of the baby (or the mother if breastfeeding) and eliminate likely irritants.

--- COMFREY & TEA TREE OIL ---

Comfrey increases the rate of cell growth, thereby speeding repair of damaged tissue. Protective, waterproof ointments or infused oils should be used for diaper rash rather than creams that soften the skin still further. Tea tree oil is added to counteract infection.

~ INGREDIENTS ~
250 g dried comfrey leaf (*Symphytum officinale*)
500 ml sunflower oil
10 ml tea tree oil (*Melaleuca alternifolia*)

~ HOW TO MAKE THE OIL ~

1 Make a hot infused oil using the comfrey and sunflower oil. For instructions, see p. 72.

2 Add the tea tree oil to the infused oil and mix well. Store in sterilized, dark glass bottles.

APPLICATION *At each diaper change, make sure the baby is well dried, using a hairdryer on a cool setting if necessary. Gently apply a little of the oil to the affected area. Leave the diaper off for a long as possible.*

Babies: Colic

The gut spasms and discomfort of colic can often be caused by rushed or tense feeding times. Check the baby's diet (or the mother's diet, if breastfeeding) to eliminate likely irritants such as hot spices, cow's milk, or wheat, and make sure that both mother and baby are relaxed and calm at meal times.

CATNIP TEA

Catnip is an ideal remedy for children – gentle and soothing, it both eases gut spasm and acts as a mild sedative encouraging sleep.

~ INGREDIENTS ~
10 g dried catnip (*Nepeta cataria*)
175 ml water

~ HOW TO MAKE THE TEA ~

Place the catnip in a teapot. Add freshly boiled water and steep for 10 minutes. Strain. The surplus can be stored in a cool place in a covered jug for up to 48 hours.

DOSAGE *Give 25–50 ml of the warm infusion before meals, reheating each dose.*

Supplementary treatments
■ If tension is a problem, nursing mothers should drink an infusion of skullcap, vervain, wood betony, or chamomile tea before feeding (to make, see p. 64).
■ Soak a compress (to make, see p. 71) in an infusion made from 15 g of chamomile flowers and 500 ml of water (to make, see p. 64) and apply to the baby's abdomen to relieve colicky pains.

Catnip tea

Babies: Teething

Teething pains can be a problem for babies from the age of 4 months (or younger in some cases).

CHAMOMILE & SAGE GUM RUB

Chamomile oil acts as a sedative while sage oil is astringent – healing, and antiseptic – helping to soothe sore gums.

~ INGREDIENTS ~
4 drops chamomile oil (*Matricaria recutita*)
2 drops sage oil (*Salvia officinalis*)
2 drops rosemary oil (*Rosmarinus officinalis*)
20 ml sunflower or sweet almond oil

~ HOW TO MAKE THE RUB ~

Pour the oils into a 50 ml sterilized, dark glass bottle and shake well.

APPLICATION *Smear a small amount of the oil on your finger and gently rub the baby's gums with it. Repeat 3 or 4 times a day.*

Supplementary treatment
■ Give 25–50 ml of a weak infusion of sedative herbs such as linden flowers or chamomile before feeds (use 10 g dried herb to 500 ml water, to make, see p. 64).

Babies: Cradle cap

Cradle cap is a scaly dermatitis that can affect the scalps of small babies and can be caused by overactive sweat glands. It is not serious or contagious.

HEARTSEASE & POT MARIGOLD OIL

Heartsease is a soothing and anti-inflammatory herb, useful for a wide range of skin disorders. Pot marigold is antifungal and astringent, encouraging healing.

~ INGREDIENTS ~
100 g pot marigold petals (*Calendula officinalis*)
150 g heartsease (*Viola tricolor*)
750 ml sunflower oil

~ HOW TO MAKE THE OIL ~

Make a hot infused oil following the instructions on p. 73.

APPLICATION *Apply a little of the oil to the affected area several times a day. Massage very gently, especially on newborn babies whose fontanelles (soft spots) have yet to close completely.*

Children: Hyperactivity

Typical symptoms of hyperactivity in children include sleeplessness, poor attention span, tearfulness, and aggressive behavior. Food intolerance or pollution are often to blame, or the child may be suffering from emotional difficulties. Check that the diet contains an adequate supply of B vitamins and minerals such as zinc and iron. Avoid all artificial colorings, preservatives, and additives, and strictly control intake of sugar, chocolate, milk, and caffeine.

Self-heal

Wood betony

—— SELF-HEAL & WOOD BETONY TEA ——

Self-heal is a common garden weed, used as a wound herb in the West. The Chinese regard it as cooling and cleansing for the liver, where pollutants and food additives tend to accumulate. Wood betony has a sedative action.

~ INGREDIENTS ~

10 g dried self-heal spikes
(*Xia Ku Cao – Prunella vulgaris*)
5 g dried wood betony (*Stachys betonica*)
5 g dried borage (*Borago officinalis*)
500 ml water
2–3 drops licorice fluid extract (*Glycyrrhiza glabra*)
or peppermint emulsion (*Mentha piperita*) per dose

~ HOW TO MAKE THE TEA ~

Place the dried herbs in a teapot and add freshly boiled water. Steep for 10 minutes and strain. The surplus can be stored in a covered jug in a cool place for up to 48 hours.

DOSAGE *Give a 100–150 ml dose for 3-to-6-year-olds 3 times a day. Flavour with licorice extract or peppermint emulsion as required (available over the counter).*

Supplementary treatments

■ Evening primrose oil can help: give 250–500 mg daily. Zinc supplements can also be useful. Give 10–20 mg daily.
■ If environmental pollution is a problem give kelp supplements, which help cleanse heavy metals from the system. Give 10–20 mg daily.

Children: Bedwetting

Regular bedwetting in young children can be the result of urinary infections, dietary deficiencies, minor physical problems with the urinary tract, or emotional upsets. Get professional advice to identify the cause.

—— CORNSILK & ST.-JOHN'S-WORT TEA ——

Cornsilk is soothing and healing for the urinary tract. St.-John's-wort is useful for anxiety and nervous tension.

~ INGREDIENTS ~

5 g dried cornsilk (*Zea mays*)
10 g dried St.-John's-wort (*Hypericum perforatum*)
500 ml water

~ HOW TO MAKE THE TEA ~

Place the dried herbs in a teapot and add freshly boiled water. Infuse for 10 minutes and strain. The surplus can be stored in a covered jug in a cool place for up to 48 hours.

DOSAGE *Give 4-year-olds a 100 ml dose 3 times a day. Increase the quantity to 150 ml for 8-year-olds.*

Supplementary treatment

■ Sweet sumach tincture is a traditional remedy for bedwetting. Give 5–10 drops in a little warm water 3 times a day (to make, see p. 68).

Children: Nits

Nits are the eggs of head lice. They spread quickly, and outbreaks in schools are commonplace. Suspect infection if children persistently scratch their heads.

—— TEA TREE RINSE ——

Tea tree oil is extracted from an Australian tree and is one of the most antiseptic and antibacterial herbs available. Unlike many oils, it does not irritate the skin.

~ INGREDIENTS ~

5 ml tea tree oil (*Melaleuca alternifolia*)
1 ml lemon oil (*Citrus limon*)
500 ml warm water

~ HOW TO MAKE THE RINSE ~

Mix the oils in a bottle and add the water. Shake well.

APPLICATION *Use as a final rinse after shampooing. Repeat each day until the infestation clears.*

Children: Threadworms

Threadworms are common in children and are highly contagious, so scrupulous hygiene is essential for the whole family. Worms lay eggs in the anus at night, so examine the child's bottom before bedtime and remove worms where possible. Worms have a life-cycle of two weeks, so treatment should be repeated after a fortnight to eliminate the problem completely.

—— CARROT & WORMWOOD MIXTURE ——

Carrot is toxic for threadworms, and in some folk traditions the child would be fed nothing but raw, grated carrot for two days to clear the problem. Wormwood also clears threadworms from the system. It has an extremely bitter taste and fennel is added to make it more palatable.

~ INGREDIENTS ~
60 ml carrot juice
10 drops wormwood tincture (*Artemisia absinthium*)
20 drops fennel tincture (*Foeniculum officinalis*)

~ HOW TO MAKE THE MIXTURE ~

Carrot juice is available commercially, or can be made using a food processor or juicer. To make the tinctures, see p. 68. Stir the tinctures into the juice. This quantity is sufficient for a single dose.

DOSAGE *Give a dose each morning before breakfast for 4 days. Repeat 2 weeks later.*

Supplementary treatments
■ Garlic is effective at clearing worms. Give 2 x 200 mg garlic capsules each morning, or finely chop a clove and mix with a little honey stirred into a cup of warm milk.
■ Cabbage is another effective remedy. Juice fresh leaves in a food processor or juicer and use 60 ml as an alternative to carrot juice in the Carrot & Wormwood Mixture.

Children: Croup

Croup usually affects children between six months and two years of age. It is caused by inflammation and obstruction of the larynx. Viral infections in the respiratory tract are generally to blame and the barking cough that results can sound quite frightening.

— *LAVENDER & EUCALYPTUS STEAMER & RUB* —

A damp, steamy atmosphere can rapidly ease symptoms. Lavender and eucalyptus oils are antiseptic and healing.

~ INGREDIENTS ~
20 drops lavender oil (*Lavandula angustifolia*)
10 drops eucalyptus oil (*Eucalyptus globulus*)
10 drops pine oil (*Pinus sylvestris*)
25 ml sweet almond or wheat germ oil

~ HOW TO APPLY THE STEAMER & RUB ~

1. Combine 10 drops of lavender, 5 drops of eucalyptus, and 5 drops of pine oil. Add to a bath of steaming water and sit the child close by until symptoms ease (do not put the child in the bath).

2. Add the same combination of oils (20 drops total) to the sweet almond or wheat germ oil and massage a little into the child's chest after the steam treatment.

CAUTION
- *Croup can be a symptom of more severe respiratory problems. Seek professional help if symptoms persist for more than 2 or 3 days or appear to be getting worse.*

Supplementary treatments
■ Give tinctures of wild cherry and white horehound (up to 5 drops of each) in a little warm water 3 times a day. To make the tinctures, see p. 68.
■ Use a humidifier in the child's room at night.

Carrot & wormwood mixture

Wormwood

Carrots

Children: Mumps

Mumps is a viral disease, affecting various glands. In children, these are generally the salivary glands in the throat, and the condition is usually mild and suitable for home treatment. Adolescents and adults should seek professional treatment, since the condition is potentially more serious, often affecting the testes.

——— *THYME & SAGE GARGLE* ———

Antiseptic gargles and mouthwashes can help combat the symptoms of mumps. Both thyme and sage are effective herbs – use either, or, as here, a mixture of the two.

~ INGREDIENTS ~
15 g dried thyme (*Thymus vulgaris*)
15 g dried sage (*Salvia officinalis*)
500 ml water

~ HOW TO MAKE THE GARGLE ~

1 Place the dried herbs in a teapot and and add freshly boiled water.

2 Steep for 15 minutes and strain. The surplus may be stored in a covered jug in a cool place or refrigerator for up to 48 hours.

DOSAGE *Use 50 ml of the infusion diluted with 50 ml of hot water as a gargle, repeating the treatment every 1–2 hours while symptoms are severe.*

Supplementary treatments
■ Follow the recommendations for fevers given on p. 87.
■ Mix 50 ml cleavers tincture and 25 ml each of echinacea and pot marigold tincture and give in 5 ml doses in warm water 3 times a day to fight infections and cleanse the lymphatic system. To make the tinctures, see p. 68.

*Thyme &
sage mouthwash*   *Sage*   *Thyme*

Children: Chickenpox

In children, chickenpox is usually a mild, if highly contagious, infection. In adults, the same virus can produce shingles. Chickenpox is characterized by rashes, which soon turn into small, red spots that blister and lead to scabs. The rashes are generally accompanied by a mild fever. Blisters are most common on the scalp, face, and body, and are very irritating. Scratching the scabs can lead to scars.

——— *BORAGE & CHICKWEED LOTION* ———

Chickweed can be used for a variety of irritant skin conditions, including eczema. Although it is often used as a cream, in this mixture it is combined with borage juice, which can also help to reduce skin irritation, to form a cooling lotion.

~ INGREDIENTS ~
10 g dried, or 30 g fresh chickweed (*Stellaria media*)
100 ml water
30 ml borage juice (*Borago officinalis*)
25 ml distilled witch hazel (*Hamamelis virginiana*)

~ HOW TO MAKE THE LOTION ~

1 Place the chickweed in a teapot and add the freshly boiled water. Steep for 15 minutes and strain.

2 Mix 45 ml of the chickweed infusion with the borage juice (available over the counter) and witch hazel in a 100 ml dark glass bottle. Shake well.

APPLICATION *Soak a cotton pad in the mixture and apply gently to the chickenpox rash, taking care not to damage the scabs. Repeat as often as necessary to soothe the irritation.*

Supplementary treatments
■ Give a cup of standard infusion of skullcap, wood betony, or chamomile 2–3 times daily as a general relaxant to calm the child (to make the infusion, see p. 64).
■ If fever is a problem, follow the recommendations given on p. 87.
■ Give 3 x 200 mg echinacea capsules or 5 ml echinacea tincture in a little warm water 3 times a day before meals. To make the capsules and tincture, see pp. 70 and 68.

Children: Whooping cough

Whooping cough often starts slowly with a mild cough and cold. Production of sticky mucus soon follows, with breathlessness, a convulsive and distressing cough, and a tendency to vomit.

CAUTION
• *Before the age of three, whooping cough can be a dangerous illness. Seek professional help in all cases.*

—— WILD LETTUCE & THYME TEA ——

Coughing spasms can be painful and exhausting. The sedative effect of wild lettuce helps to calm the child, while thyme is antiseptic and combines with other expectorants in the mix to help clear the mucus. This tea can form a useful adjunct to professional treatments.

~ INGREDIENTS ~
5 g dried elecampane root (*Inula helenium*)
5 g licorice root (*Glycyrrhiza glabra*)
750 ml water
10 g dried wild lettuce (*Lactuca virosa*)
5 g dried thyme (*Thymus vulgaris*)
10 g dried mullein flowers (*Verbascum thapsus*)

~ HOW TO MAKE THE TEA ~
1. Put the elecampane, licorice and water in a pan and simmer for 20 minutes to make a decoction.

2. Mix the remaining dried herbs in a teapot and pour on the simmering decoction. Infuse for 10 minutes and strain.

DOSAGE *Give a large mugful up to 6 times a day.*

Supplementary treatments
■ Make sure the child's room is well ventilated and dry.
■ Mix 2 ml each of hyssop, cypress, and basil oil in 50 ml of sweet almond oil. Rub on to the child's chest 2 or 3 times a day. Alternatively, put the undiluted essential oils into a vaporizer or diffuser in the child's room at night.
■ Give 3 x 200 mg echinacea capsules twice a day if the child can swallow them. If not, give 5 ml echinacea tincture in warm water twice daily. To make, see pp. 70 and 68.

—— Other Childhood Ailments ——

See also the following ailments in the adult section: constipation p. 104; diarrhea p. 105; earache p. 91; gastritis p. 106, and nausea & vomiting p. 107.
Note: See p. 128 for advice on reducing adult dosages to suit children.

Hyssop

Marshmallow

Hyssop & marshmallow infusion

Children: Measles

Measles is a highly contagious viral disease, characterized by a heavy cold, harsh, dry cough, a blotchy rash that usually starts behind the ears, and bloodshot, light-sensitive eyes. It usually occurs in local epidemics, and complications include pneumonia and middle ear infections. In many cases it is important to seek professional help.

—— HYSSOP & MARSHMALLOW INFUSION ——

Relaxing expectorants help to soothe the coughing associated with measles. Hyssop is an ideal expectorant for children and marshmallow is a demulcent, helping to lubricate the mucous membranes.

~ INGREDIENTS ~
30 g dried hyssop (*Hyssopus officinalis*)
30 g dried marshmallow leaf (*Althaea officinalis*)
30 g dried ribwort plantain (*Plantago major*)
water
2 ml licorice fluid extract per dose (*Glycyrrhiza glabra*)

~ HOW TO MAKE THE INFUSION ~
Mix the herbs and store in an airtight container. Place a teaspoon of the mixture in a tisane cup or small teapot and add freshly boiled water. Infuse for 10 minutes and strain.

DOSAGE *Give a teacup dose 4 times a day, before meals and at night, adding the licorice fluid extract as a flavoring.*

Supplementary treatments
■ Follow the recommendations for fever on p. 87.
■ Give 3 x 200 mg echinacea capsules or 5 ml echinacea tincture 3 times daily. To make, see pp. 70 and 68.
■ Use well-strained eyebright or self-heal infusions in an eyebath to soothe irritation. To use, see p. 79.

ROADSIDE REMEDIES

"ALL NATURE," WROTE the sixteenth-century herbalist Paracelsus, "is like one single apothecary's shop, covered only with the roof of heaven. . ." In an emergency outdoors, wild plants can provide help until more conventional remedies are available. However, as Paracelsus also pointed out, "In all things there is a poison and there is nothing without poison – it depends only upon the dose whether a poison is poison or not. . ." Some healing plants have a nastier side to them and careful handling is required – especially if small children are around.

Shepherd's purse aerial parts

Wild herbs

The following may be gathered for use in homemade remedies, and many of them are useful in emergency first aid – when minor accidents happen on country walks and the first aid box is out of reach.

SHEPHERD'S PURSE (*Capsella bursa-pastoris*) stops bleeding. Use fresh in a poultice on cuts and scrapes.

MARSH WOUNDWORT (*Stachys palustris*), also called all-heal, was once used as a poultice on very severe injuries. Use the bruised leaves on minor cuts. The juice may be taken internally for diarrhea.

—————— CAUTIONS ——————
- *Use a botanical field guide to identify plants correctly.*
- *The remedies listed here are for emergency use or for minor problems. Seek medical help for serious cuts, burns, and sprains as soon as possible – an antitetanus injection may be recommended.*

Marsh woundwort flowering spikes

BEAR'S BREECHES (*Acanthus mollis*) Apply the crushed leaves to minor burns and scalds.
BUTTER-AND-EGGS (*Linaria vulgaris*) Make a poultice with fresh leaves to treat cuts or hemorrhoids. A well-strained infusion can be an effective eye wash for sore eyes.
COMMON MALLOW (*Malva sylvestris*) The leaves and flowers can be used as a poultice for wounds.
CORNFLOWER (*Centaurea cyanus*) Bathe sore eyes with a well-strained infusion.
CREEPING JENNY (*Lysimachia nummularia*) A poultice of fresh leaves or a compress made from a strong infusion can be used to treat wounds and sores.
HERB BENNET (*Geum urbanum*) Chew the clove-flavored root to sweeten the breath. A decoction can ease chills and diarrhea.

GARLIC MUSTARD (*Alliaria petiolata*) Also known as Jack-by-the-hedge. The fresh leaves can be crushed and applied to insect bites to relieve itching.
MEADOWSWEET (*Filipendula ulmaria*) Commonly found in wayside ditches; use the infusion to settle stomach upsets.
PURPLE LOOSESTRIFE (*Lythrum salicaria*) The infusion may be taken for diarrhea or used in compresses to help ease skin rashes.
STINGING NETTLE (*Urtica dioica*) Use the infusion in compresses for eczema, as a gargle for sore throats and mouth ulcers, or on cotton swabs to stop nosebleeds.
WHITE DEADNETTLE (*Lamium album*) The infusion may be taken internally for cystitis or used in a compress to treat hemorrhoids.

YARROW (*Achillea millefolium*) is a useful wound herb. Use as a fresh poultice or insert a leaf in the nostrils to stop nosebleeds.

Yarrow aerial parts

DAISY (*Bellis perennis*) was once known as bruisewort. A poultice of the fresh plant or a compress soaked in an infusion can relieve bruises and sprains.

Daisy plant

Herb Robert aerial parts

SELF HEAL (*Prunella vulgaris*) is astringent and healing for mouth ulcers, hemorrhoids, and sores. The infusion also makes a useful eyewash for sore or irritated eyes.

Flowering self-heal

HERB ROBERT (*Geranium robertianum*) is an astringent herb for cuts and scrapes and was once thought capable of repairing broken bones. Use an infusion for sore throats, mouth ulcers, and eye inflammations. The crushed leaves are said to keep mosquitoes away.

DOCK (*Rumex obtusifolius*) is a well known antidote to nettle stings. Rub a freshly crushed leaf over the affected area.

Dock leaf

Common plantain leaves

COMMON PLANTAIN (*Plantago major*) makes a readily available remedy for insect bites and stings. Rub the fresh leaves on to the affected part.

Handle with care

Some plants and flowers are highly toxic. Borage, chamomile, hops, primulas, runner beans, and yarrow can cause rashes. Holly, laburnum, mistletoe, privet, spindle, sweet pea, and white bryony have toxic fruits. If a child is ill after eating a plant, take a sample with you to the hospital.

- **Deadly nightshade** (*Atropa belladonna*) is used by herbalists as a sedative and antispasmodic, but the black berries are fatal.
- **Greater celandine** (*Chelidonium majus*) has a yellow sap that clears warts, but can irritate healthy skin. Handle with care.
- **Hemlock** (*Conium maculatum*) is easily mistaken for cow parsley or sweet cicely: look for leaf textures, smell, seed shapes, and red blotches on the stem. Do not swallow (this can be fatal); handle with care.
- **Henbane** (*Hyoscyamus niger*) is used medicinally to treat asthma and colic. It is reasonably safe to handle, but do not swallow the fresh plant.
- **Monkshood** (*Aconitum napellus*) is poisonous and touching it can cause numbness.
- **Rue** (*Ruta graveolens*) is edible, but on sunny days, sap and damp leaves can cause a rash.

THE HERBAL FIRST AID KIT

MOST HOUSEHOLDS HAVE their regular stock of over-the-counter pharmaceuticals for emergencies, but herbal alternatives can be just as effective, often offering more healing properties from a small number of basic ingredients. The kitchen cupboard can also be useful, providing garlic, ginger, tea, honey, and other ingredients. Supplement these household items with over-the-counter herbal preparations.

FIRST AID KIT
Keep the first aid kit easily accessible, but out of the reach of children.

ARNICA CREAM
Effective for bruises and sprains. Do not use on broken skin.

CHICKWEED CREAM
Valuable for drawing splinters, boils, and insect stings or for easing burns, scalds, and eczema.

ALOE VERA
To soothe minor burns, scalds, or sunburn, break off a leaf from an aloe plant, split it open, and apply the thick gel to the affected area.

MARIGOLD CREAM
Often sold as calendula; an antiseptic and antifungal cream, used for cuts, scrapes, and dry skin.

GARLIC
Rub fresh cloves on acne and other infected spots. Use crushed garlic to draw corns. Take internally for chest infections and thrush.

TEA TREE OIL
One of the most antiseptic and antifungal oils; use for cuts and scrapes as well as on warts and cold sores.

HOMEOPATHIC ARNICA 6X
Essential for domestic shocks or accidents, one tablet should be taken at 30 minute intervals until the patient feels calmer and more settled.

HONEY
Draws pus and poisons out of wounds. Useful for colds, mixed with hot lemon juice and water.

DISTILLED WITCH HAZEL
Use for minor burns and sunburn. Soak a swab in witch hazel to stop bleeding. Frozen witch hazel soothes insect bites, varicose veins, and bruises. Keep a clearly labeled ice cube tray of witch hazel in the freezer.

RESCUE REMEDY
The Bach Flower Remedies have a potent effect on the emotions. Rescue Remedy is an excellent emergency treatment for shocks and nervous upsets. Take 2–3 drops undiluted on the tongue.

EVENING PRIMROSE OIL
A useful hangover cure, restoring liver function. Take a large dose (2–3 g) "the morning after" for rapid relief.

LAVENDER OIL
Dilute 2–3 drops in a teaspoon of sweet almond oil and use to massage the temples and neck for tension headaches and migraine. Use the same mix for burns and scalds.

SLIPPERY ELM TABLETS
Take 1–2 x 200 g capsules for indigestion, gastritis, and stomach upsets, to line the stomach and reduce inflammation.

ECHINACEA CAPSULES
A valuable standby for colds and flu. Take 2 x 200 g capsules or tablets 3 times a day at the first hint of infection.

Chamomile   *Peppermint*

DRIED HERBS
Keep an assortment of dried herbs or herbal teabags handy for infusions. Use chamomile flowers for shock, nervous upsets, insomnia, or indigestion; fennel or peppermint for indigestion; lavender for headaches and migraines; vervain for stress and digestive problems, and elderflower for phlegm.

Herbs for holidays

Holidays can be easily spoiled by minor ailments. Basic hygiene rules are essential in exotic locations: peel fruit and do not eat any other raw foods, and do not drink tapwater or have ice cubes in drinks. If stomach upsets and diarrhea occur, try eating papaya – a traditional remedy in many tropical areas – or drink strong black tea without milk or sugar. Take a holiday first aid kit to cope with other problems.

FIRST AID CHECKLIST

• Cuts and scrapes: tea tree oil or pot marigold cream. Dab a little on to the affected part.
• Diarrhea: mix equal amounts of bistort, honeysuckle, and marshmallow tinctures. Take 5 ml in warm water every 2–3 hours.
• Heatstroke: sugar and salt. Take ½ a teaspoon of each in some water.
• Insect bites, cuts, and scrapes: use 2–3 drops of lemon balm oil in a teaspoon of sweet almond oil or St.-John's-wort and marigold tinctures. Dab onto the affected part.
• Jet lag: Siberian ginseng or chamomile teabags.
• Shock: Take a homeopathic *Arnica* 6x pill at 30 minute intervals.
• Sprains and bruises: arnica or comfrey cream (do not use on broken skin).
• Stomach upsets: meadowsweet tincture. Take 5 ml in warm water 3–4 times a day. Chamomile or peppermint teabags are also useful.
• Sunburn: 5 ml lavender oil combined with 20 ml infused St.-John's-wort oil. Dab on the skin.
• Travel sickness and vomiting: crystallized ginger or ginger capsules.

St.-John's-wort & lavender oil   *Tea tree oil*   *St.-John's-wort & marigold tincture*   *Meadowsweet tincture*   *Honeysuckle, bistort & marshmallow tincture*

Arnica 6x tablets   *Crystallized ginger*   *Arnica cream*   *Herbal teabags*

OTHER MEDICINAL HERBS

Each entry gives the common name, botanical name, parts used and their actions.
Caution: do not take essential oils internally except when directed to do so by a professional practitioner.

ANGELICA: *Angelica archangelica*
Leaves: carminative, antispasmodic, diaphoretic, expectorant, diuretic, digestive tonic, antirheumatic, uterine stimulant. **Caution:** avoid large doses in pregnancy and in diabetes.

ANISE: *Pimpinella anisum*
Essential oil, seeds: expectorant, carminative, antiseptic, antispasmodic.

ASHWAGANDHA: *Withania somnifera*
Root: tonic, aphrodisiac, sedative, astringent, nervine.

BAI SHAO, WHITE PEONY:
Paeonia lactiflora
Root: antibacterial, reduces blood pressure, antispasmodic, anti-inflammatory, analgesic, tranquilizing.

BAI ZHI: *Atractylodes macrocephala*
Rhizome: digestive tonic, diuretic, lowers blood sugar levels.

BASIL: *Ocimum basilicum*
Leaves, essential oil: antidepressant, antiseptic, stimulating, soothing, prevents vomiting, carminative, febrifuge, tonic. **Caution:** avoid essential oil in pregnancy.

BAYBERRY: *Myrica cerifera*
Bark: stimulant, astringent, diaphoretic.

BEARBERRY, UVA-URSI:
Arctostaphylos uva-ursi
Leaves: astringent, urinary antiseptic. **Caution:** high doses may cause nausea.

BENZOIN: *Styrax benzoin*
Essential oil, gum: expectorant, astringent, antispasmodic.

BISTORT: *Polygonum bistorta*
Root: astringent, decongestant, styptic.

BLACK HAW: *Viburnum prunifolium*
Root, bark: antispasmodic, sedative, astringent, relaxant, tonic, uterine relaxant, anti-inflammatory.

BLACK HOREHOUND: *Ballota nigra*
Aerial parts: prevents vomiting, stimulant, tonic.

BLUE FLAG: *Iris versicolor*
Rhizome: anti-inflammatory, stimulant, diuretic.

BOGBEAN: *Menyanthes trifoliata*
Leaves: antirheumatic, bitter, tonic.

BOLDO: *Peumus boldo*
Leaves: liver stimulant, diuretic.

BONESET: *Eupatorium perfoliatum*
Aerial parts: diaphoretic, laxative, antispasmodic, expectorant.
Caution: high doses can cause vomiting.

BORAGE: *Borago officinalis*
Leaves, flowers: adrenal stimulants, diuretic, promotes lactation, febrifuge, antirheumatic, diaphoretic, expectorant. **Seed oil:** a source of gamma-linolenic acid.
Note: restricted herb in Australia and New Zealand.

BUCKWHEAT:
Fagopyrum esculentum
Leaves: reduce blood pressure, repairs blood vessels.

BU GU ZHI: *Psoralea corylifolia*
Fruit: diuretic, astringent, antibacterial, kidney tonic.
Caution: can cause photosensitivity of the skin.

CABBAGE: *Brassica oleracea*
Leaves: anti-inflammatory, anti-bacterial, liver decongestant.

CAJEPUT: *Melaleuca leucadendra*
Essential oil: diaphoretic, expectorant, aromatic.

CAMPHOR: *Cinnamomum camphora*
Gum oil: carminative, analgesic, antiseptic, sedative, stimulant.

CARAWAY: *Carum carvi*
Seeds: digestive stimulant, antiseptic.

CASCARA: *Rhamnus purshiana*
Bark: digestive tonic, laxative.
Caution: avoid in pregnancy.

CATNIP: *Nepeta cataria*
Aerial parts: antispasmodic, carminative, digestive stimulant, diaphoretic.

CHASTE-TREE: *Vitex agnus-castus*
Berries: hormone stimulant.
Caution: high doses may cause formication (a sensation of ants crawling on the skin).

CHICKWEED: *Stellaria media*
Aerial parts: astringent, antirheumatic, heals wounds, demulcent.

CHINESE CHRYSANTHEMUM *see*
JU HUA

CLARY: *Salvia sclarea*
Essential oil: carminative, nerve tonic, uterine stimulant.
Cautions: high doses are toxic and may cause headaches. Avoid in pregnancy.

CLOVE: *Syzygium aromaticum*
Essential oil, flower buds: carminative, antispasmodic, prevents vomiting. **Caution:** do not exceed stated dose.

COMFREY: *Symphytum officinale*
Aerial parts, root: cell proliferator, astringent, heals wounds, demulcent, expectorant.
Cautions: avoid excessive internal consumption of the herb. Use only on clean wounds.
Note: restricted herb in Australia and New Zealand.

COUCHGRASS: *Agropyron repens*
Rhizome: cleansing diuretic, demulcent.

COWSLIP: *Primula veris*
Flowers: sedative nervine, calming, astringent, promotes sweating. **Root:** stimulating, expectorant, astringent, diaphoretic. **Cautions:** avoid if aspirin-sensitive or if taking blood-thinning drugs. Do not take high doses in pregnancy.

CRAMP BARK: *Viburnum opulus*
Bark: antispasmodic, sedative, astringent, muscle relaxant, cardiac tonic, uterine relaxant, anti-inflammatory.

CRANESBILL: *Geranium maculatum*
Leaves, root: astringent.

CYPRESS: *Cupressus sempervirens*

Essential oil: antiseptic, sedative.

DAMIANA: *Turnera diffusa*
Aerial parts: aphrodisiac, diuretic, urinary antiseptic, laxative, nervine.

DANG SHEN: *Codonopsis pilosula*
Root: demulcent, expectorant, tonic.

DEVIL'S CLAW: *Harpagophytum procumbens*
Tuber: diuretic, anti-inflammatory, antirheumatic, analgesic, sedative, liver stimulant.

DILL: *Anethum graveolens*
Seeds: carminative.

ELECAMPANE: *Inula helenium*
Root, flowers: tonic, stimulating expectorant, diaphoretic, antibacterial, antifungal, antiparasitic, digestive stimulant.

EPHEDRA *see* **MA HUANG**

FALSE UNICORN ROOT, HELONIAS:
Chamaelirium luteum
Rhizome: diuretic, emetic, uterine tonic.

FENUGREEK: *Trigonella foenum-graecum*
Seeds: digestive tonic, anti-inflammatory, promote milk flow, locally demulcent, uterine stimulant, reduces blood sugar levels, aphrodisiac. **Aerial parts:** antispasmodic. **Cautions:** avoid in pregnancy. The aerial parts may be used in labor. Insulin-dependent diabetics should avoid unless under professional guidance.

FIGWORT: *Scrophularia nodosa*
Aerial parts: diuretic, laxative, heart stimulant, circulatory stimulant, anti-inflammatory.
Caution: avoid in cases of abnormally rapid heartbeat.

FORSYTHIA *see* **Lian Qiao**

FRANKINCENSE: *Boswellia thurifera*
Gum: antiseptic, tonic, astringent, carminative.

FUMITORY: *Fumaria officinalis*

Aerial parts: antispasmodic, liver and gall bladder stimulant.

GAN CAO *Glycyrrhiza uralensis*
Root: diaphoretic, antirheumatic, analgesic, antispasmodic.

GENTIAN: *Gentiana lutea*
Root: digestive stimulant, sedative, anti-inflammatory, febrifuge.

GINKGO: *Ginkgo biloba*
Leaves: relax blood vessels, circulatory stimulant.

GOAT'S RUE: *Galega officinalis*
Aerial parts: antispasmodic, stimulant. **Caution**: diabetics should avoid unless under professional guidance.

GOLDEN ROD: *Solidago virgaurea*
Aerial parts: decongestant, diaphoretic, anti-inflammatory, urinary antiseptic, sedative, reduces blood pressure.

GOTU KOLA: *Centella asiatica*
Aerial parts: diuretic, sedating nervine, cooling, tonic. **Caution**: high doses can cause headaches or aggravate itching.

GOU QI ZI: *Lycium chinense*
Berries: antitussive, lowers blood pressure, lowers cholesterol.

GRAVELROOT:
Eupatorium purpureum
Root: diuretic, antirheumatic, encourages menstruation.

GROUND IVY: *Glechoma hederacea*
Leaves: astringent, decongestant.

GUARANA: *Paullinia cupana*
Seeds: stimulant, astringent.

HAWTHORN: *Crataegus oxyacantha*
Flowering tops, berries: relaxant, cardiac tonic, astringent.

HELONIAS *see* **FALSE UNICORN ROOT**

HOPS: *Humulus lupulus*
Strobiles: sedative, male anaphrodisiac, nerve tonic, bitter digestive stimulant, diuretic. **Cautions**: do not exceed the stated dose. Avoid in depression. The growing plant can cause skin rashes.

HORSETAIL: *Equisetum arvense*
Aerial parts: astringent, stops bleeding, diuretic, anti-inflammatory, tissue healer.

ISPHAGULA, PSYLLIUM SEEDS:
Plantago ovata
Seeds: demulcent, laxative.

JU HUA, CHINESE CHRYSANTHEMUM:
Chrysanthemum morifolium
Flowers: anti-inflammatory, antimicrobial, lowers blood pressure.

LADY'S MANTLE: *Alchemilla vulgaris*
Aerial parts: astringent, menstrual regulator, digestive tonic, anti-inflammatory. **Caution**: avoid in pregnancy.

LESSER CELANDINE *see* **PILEWORT**

LIAN QIAO, FORSYTHIA:
Forsythia suspensa
Fruit: antibacterial, anti-inflammatory, antirheumatic, circulatory stimulant. **Caution**: avoid in diarrhea.

LING ZHI: *Ganoderma lucidem*
Fruiting body: immune stimulant, nervine, tonic, antitussive, anti-allergenic, anti-bacterial.

LINSEED: *Linum usitatissimum*
Seeds: demulcent, soothing, anti-tussive, antiseptic, anti-inflammatory, laxative. **Cautions**: Do not drink artists' linseed oil. Do not exceed the stated dose.

LUNGWORT: *Pulmonaria officinalis*
Flowering plant: soothing expectorant, astringent, styptic.

MAGNOLIA *see* **XIN YIN HUA**

MA HUANG, EPHEDRA:
Ephedra sinica
Twigs: febrifuge, antispasmodic, diaphoretic, diuretic, antibacterial. **Cautions**: restricted herb in the UK, for use by professional practitioners only. Restricted herb in Australia and New Zealand. Not to be used if taking MAO inhibitors as antidepressants. Should be avoided in cases of glaucoma, hypertension, and coronary thrombosis.

MARJORAM: *Origanum marjorana*
Leaves, essential oil: stimulant, promotes menstruation, antispasmodic, diaphoretic.

MILK THISTLE: *Carduus marianus*
Seeds: liver stimulant and tonic, promote milk flow, demulcent, antidepressant.

MOTHERWORT: *Leonurus cardiaca*
Aerial parts: uterine stimulant, relaxant, cardiac tonic, carminative. **Caution**: avoid in pregnancy; safe in labor.

MUGWORT: *Artemisia vulgaris*
Aerial parts: bitter digestive tonic, stimulant, stimulating nervine, menstrual regulator, anti-rheumatic. **Cautions**: avoid in pregnancy and if breastfeeding.

MULLEIN: *Verbascum thapsus*
Flowers, leaves: expectorant, mild diuretic, demulcent, sedative, heal wounds, astringent, anti-inflammatory.

MYRRH: *Commiphora molmol*
Resin, essential oil: antifungal, antiseptic, astringent, bitter, expectorant, circulatory stimulant, decongestant. **Caution**: avoid in pregnancy.

NUTMEG: *Myristica fragrans*
Kernel, essential oil: carminative, digestive stimulant, antispasmodic, prevents vomiting, appetite stimulant, anti-inflammatory. **Cautions**: large doses (7.5 g or more in a single dose) are dangerous, producing convulsions and palpitations. Avoid in pregnancy.

NU ZHEN ZI: *Ligustrum lucidum*
Berries: tonic, immunostimulant, diuretic.

OATS: *Avena sativa*
Grain: antidepressant, restorative nerve tonic, nutritive. **Oatbran**: antithrombotic, reduces blood cholesterol levels. **Caution**: those sensitive to gluten must allow the decoction or tincture to settle, then decant the clear liquid only for use.

PAPAYA: *Carica papaya*
Fruit: rich in vitamins, digestive remedy, anti-allergenic, wound herb.

PASSIONFLOWER: *Passiflora incarnata*
Leaves: sedative, anodyne, hypnotic, antispasmodic. **Caution**: avoid high doses in pregnancy.

PATCHOULI: *Pogostemon cablin*
Essential oil: antidepressant, aphrodisiac, sedative, tonic, antiseptic.

PELLITORY-OF-THE-WALL:
Parietaria diffusa
Aerial parts: demulcent, diuretic.

PILEWORT, LESSER CELANDINE:
Ranunculus ficaria
Root, leaves: astringent.

PINE: *Pinus sylvestris*
Essential oil: expectorant, antiseptic, decongestant, rubefacient.

PLEURISY ROOT: *Asclepias tuberosa*
Root: expectorant, carminative, laxative, relaxes peripheral blood vessels.

PRICKLY ASH:
Zanthoxylum americanum
Bark: carminative, circulatory stimulant, promotes sweating, tonic.

PSYLLIUM SEEDS *see* **ISPHAGULA**

RAMPS: *Allium tricoccum*
Aerial parts, bulbs: decrease blood sugar levels, lower cholesterol, antimicrobial, tonic.

RASPBERRY: *Rubus idaeus*
Leaves: astringent, preparative for childbirth, stimulant, digestive tonic. **Berries**: diuretic, laxative, diaphoretic, cleansing. **Caution**: avoid high doses of the leaves during early pregnancy.

RED CLOVER: *Trifolium pratense*
Flowers: cleansing, antispasmodic, diuretic, anti-inflammatory, possible estrogenic activity.

RHUBARB: *Rheum palmatum*
Root: laxative, digestive tonic, astringent, antibacterial. **Cautions**: avoid in pregnancy, gout and arthritic conditions. The leaves are toxic.

ROSE: *Rosa* spp
Essential oil: antidepressant, antispasmodic, sedative, aphrodisiac, cleansing, expectorant, antibacterial, antiviral, antiseptic, kidney tonic, blood tonic, menstrual regulator, anti-inflammatory. **Cautions**: only use the best quality oil medicinally. Only take internally under professional supervision.

SANDALWOOD: *Santalum album*
Essential oil: antidepressant, antiseptic, antispasmodic, carminative, expectorant.

SAW PALMETTO: *Serenoa repens*
Berries: aphrodisiac, diuretic, sedative.

SELF-HEAL: *Prunella vulgaris*
Aerial parts: antibacterial, reduces blood pressure, diuretic, astringent, heals wounds. **Flower spikes**: liver

stimulant, reduce blood pressure, antibacterial.

SENNA: *Cassia senna*
Leaves, fruits: stimulating, laxative. **Caution:** avoid in pregnancy, unless prescribed by professional practitioner.

SHU DI HUANG:
Rehmannia glutinosa
Prepared root: demulcent, laxative, styptic, blood tonic.

SLIPPERY ELM: *Ulmus fulva*
Bark: demulcent, nutritive, astringent.

SOAP BARK: *Quillaja saponaria*
Inner bark: detergent, expectorant, anti-inflammatory. **Caution:** do not take internally.

SUNDEW: *Drosera rotundifolia*
Flowering plant: relaxant expectorant, antispasmodic, demulcent.

SWEET SUMACH: *Rhus aromatica*
Root, bark: astringent, diuretic, antidiabetic.

TEA: *Camellia sinensis*
Leaves: stimulant, astringent, antibacterial, diuretic.

THUJA: *Thuja occidentalis*
Leaf tips: astringent, antimicrobial, anti-inflammatory, muscle stimulant. **Caution:** avoid in pregnancy.

TORMENTIL: *Potentilla erecta*
Root: astringent, promotes healing.

UVA-URSI *see* **BEARBERRY**

VALERIAN: *Valeriana officinalis*
Root: tranquilizing, antispasmodic, expectorant, diuretic, reduces blood pressure, carminative, mild anodyne. **Cautions:** do not take for more than 2–3 weeks without a break. Avoid if taking sleep-inducing drugs.

WHITE DEADNETTLE:
Lamium album
Flowering tops: astringent, tonic for reproductive organs, antispasmodic.

WHITE HOREHOUND:
Marrubium vulgare
Aerial parts: antispasmodic, bitter, stimulating expectorant, soothing tonic.

WHITE PEONY *see* **BAI SHAO**

WILD CHERRY: *Prunus serotina*
Bark: antitussive, digestive stimulant, sedative. **Cautions:** avoid in acute infections. Can cause drowsiness.

WILLOW: *Salix alba*
Bark, leaves: antirheumatic, antiseptic, anti-inflammatory, analgesic, astringent, bitter digestive tonic.

WITCH HAZEL:
Hamamelis virginiana
Bark, leaves: astringent, hemostatic. **Cautions:** use externally only.

WORMWOOD: *Artemezia absinthium*
Aerial parts: bitter digestive tonic, uterine stimulant, antibiotic, bile stimulant, carminative, antiseptic. **Caution:** avoid if pregnant or breastfeeding.

XIN YIN HUA, MAGNOLIA:
Magnolia liliflora
Flower, flowerbuds: decongestant, antifungal, analgesic, anti-inflammatory. **Cautions:** high doses can cause dizziness.

YLANG YLANG: *Cananga odorata*
Essential oil: antidepressant, antiseptic, aphrodisiac, sedative. **Caution:** use sparingly, excess can cause headaches and nausea.

Glossary

Analgesic: relieves pain.
Anodyne: allays pain.
Antispasmodic: reduces muscle spasm and tension.
Antitussive: inhibits coughing reflex.
Aperient: mild laxative.
Bitter: stimulates secretion of digestive juices, stimulates appetite.
Carminative: relieves gas; digestive colic.
Demulcent: soothes damaged or inflamed surfaces.
Diaphoretic: promotes sweating.
Diuretic: encourages urine flow.
Febrifuge: reduces fever.
Mucilage: soft, slippery substances that protect mucous membranes.
Nervine: affects the nervous system.
Rubefacient: stimulates blood flow to the skin.
Saponins: plant substance similar to soap; expectorant.
Styptic: stops external bleeding.
Systemic: affecting the entire body.
Tonify: strengthen and restore.
Topical: local adminstration of a remedy, e.g. to the skin.
Yang: associated with male energy – dry, hot.
Yin: associated with female energy – damp, cold.

Consulting a Herbalist & Addresses

Many people regularly use herbs as safe and effective home remedies for minor ailments, but persistent or serious problems need help from a qualified herbal practitioner. Choosing someone who you can trust can be just as important as taking the most appropriate herbs. The best way to find a practitioner is through personal recommendation from a like-minded friend.

Some herbalists follow an orthodox path, prescribing herbal remedies to ease symptoms, while others focus on holistic treatments urging major lifestyle changes.

A first consultation takes about an hour, and subsequent ones about 20 minutes or so. Simple on-site tests may include urine analysis or measuring hemoglobin levels from a tiny drop of blood. Herbalists look into a patient's medical history as well as reviewing the current illness, asking about allergies, family tendencies, diet, lifestyle, stresses, and worries.

At the end of the consultation, the herbalist makes up a prescription, based on tinctures, creams, oils, capsules, or dried herbs. Whatever the remedy, healing is a two-way process and patients must take the responsibility for their own health and actively participate in any cure.

American Association of Acupuncture and Oriental Medicine
433 Front Street
Catasawqua, PA 18032
(610) 433-2448

American Asociation of Oriental Healing Arts
P.O. Box 718, Jamaica Plains, MA 02130   (617) 236-5867

American Botanical Council
P.O. Box 210660, Austin, TX 78720
(512) 331-8868

American Herbal Products Association
P.O. Box 2410, Austin, TX 78768
(512) 320-8555

Common Sense
109 Lincoln Ave., Rutland, UT 05701
(802) 773-0582

National Health Federation
P.O. Box 688, Monrovia, CA 91017
(800) 643-4968

The American Herbalists' Guild
P.O. Box 1683, Soquel, CA 95073
(408) 464-2441

The Herb Research Foundation
1007 Pearl Street, Suite 200, Boulder, CO 808302

Herbal Suppliers

Aphrodisia
264 Bleeker Street, New York NY 10014
(212) 989-6004

Herbs Products Co.
11012 Magnolia Blvd., North Hollywood, CA 91601
(818) 984–3141

May Way Trading Chinese Herb Company
1338 Cypress Street, Oakland, CA 94607
(510) 208-3113

Kiehls Pharmacy
109 Third Avenue, New York, NY 10009 (*essential oils*)

Milan Home Wine and Beer
57 Spring Street, NY 10012
(*winepresses, spices, vinegar*)

INDEX

NOTE: Page numbers in **bold** refer to main herb entries in the *A-to-Z of Medicinal Herbs* and *Other Medicinal Herbs*.

Author's Acknowledgments
Like enthusiastic cooks, medical herbalists endlessly collect and
adapt ideas for using herbs, as well as "recipes" for creams,
syrups or lotions, from friends and colleagues. My thanks are
therefore due to many fellow herbalists who have generously
shared their knowledge with me over very many years. It
would be impossible to list everyone – it may read like the
membership roll of the NIMH – but especial love and
gratitude to Andrew Chevallier, Stephen and Carol Church,
Carole Guyett, Christopher Hedley, Rowan Stainton, Dragana
Carter and Anne Warren-Davis.

Publisher's Acknowledgments
Dorling Kindersley would like to thank: Peter Allen (*Ugly*
modeling agency), Jane, Stephen, Charlotte and William Bull,
Thomas Greene, Mary Ody, Hossein Razazan, Nicki Sarluis,
Kate Scott, Susan Swaris and Tina Vaughan for modeling;
Ellen Cramer (*Artistic Licence* agency) for make up; Stephen
Bull for collecting herb specimens; Rosemary Titterington at
Iden Croft Herbs and Chelsea Physic Garden; Helen Barnett,
Antonia Cunningham, Charlotte Evans, Nell Graville, Valerie
Horn, Colin Nicholls and Nick Turpin for editorial assistance;
and Sarah Ereira for compiling the index.

Photography Credits
key to picture positions: t=top b=bottom r=right l=left c=center

All photography by Steve Gorton except:
Peter Anderson: 40 tr; 44 bc, br. Martin Cameron: 55; 56 (tl, tr, br);
57; 63 bl, br; 68 (except tr) 70 t,l; 71 tl, tr, bl, br; 72 (except tr); 73 (except
tl); 75 bl; 76 bl, br. Andy Crawford: 53 b, r; 63 tc, tr; 66-7; 68 tr; 69 br;
70 b; 71 bc; 72 tr; 74; 75 (except bl); 76 tl, tc, tr; 77; 78-9. Nigel Fletcher
and Matthew Ward: 20 t; 31 tr; 33 bl; 34 c; 35 tr; 36 bc; 39 br; 46 bl; 95 bl.
Dave King: 2-3; 5 tl, br; 8-9; 10 bl-br; 12 b (except br); 14 bl-br; 16 bl-br;
17; 18 b (except left oil); 20 b (except br); 22 b (except br); 24 bl-br;
26 bl-br; 28-9; 37 tc; 39 tl; 40 br, bc; 41 bl; 42 c; 43 r; 48-9; 52
(except widger); 56 bl; 58-9; 62; 64-5; 80-1; 82-3; 84-5; 102-3 tc; 145.
David Murray: 38 l. National Trust Photographic Library/Mike Williams:
50. Martin Norris: 136 tl, tc. Tim Ridley: 12 br; 18 bc (oil); 20 br, 22 br.
Steve Shott: 11. Clive Streeter: 31 bl; 33 tl; 43 tl; 60-1; 86; 88; 92-3; 103
(dried bistort root); 104-5; 106-7; 111; 134; 135 t, cr, br.
Matthew Ward: 115 lc.